JOE HAMMOND was a critically acclaimed writer and playwright. He took part in the Royal Court Studio Writers' Group in 2012, having previously been mentored by the theatre and the BBC. His debut London production 'Where the Mangrove Grows' played at Theatre503 in 2012 and was later published by Bloomsbury. His memoir, *A Short History of Falling*, chronicling the last days of his life, was published by 4th Estate in 2019 shortly before his death. He lived in Hampshire with his wife and two sons.

Praise for *A Short History of Falling*:

'It is unforgettable: powerful, moving and life changing. Joe Hammond shows us how great beauty can be found in the darkest of situations'   Russell Tovey

'Joe's raw and honest depiction of his condition will leave you with a new-found wonder for the human body . . . Joe's words paint such a vivid picture of his experiences that it's like you're there with him, for every fall, every laugh, every quiet thought'
                                        The Marie Curie Trust

'He approaches his plight with a curiosity that rises above self-pity . . . Although he can no longer take part in family life as he once did, he never disappears into illness (as many do). And the book itself keeps him connected. What one notices throughout is the ascendancy of the writing: fit and unaffected and strong. And the images he alights upon are brilliant – there is a gallantry to them . . . At every turn, his witty precision deepens the narrative's impact . . . It is a moving reiteration that a "short" history is our human lot'   *Observer*

'A beautifully written reminder that life can be tragic as well as full of joy'
  Christie Watson, author of *The Language of Kindness*

'I loved this book, and read it in a day. It's surprising and uncommon and I don't think I'll ever forget it'
  Sunjeev Sahota, author of *The Year of the Runaways*

'His voice is captivating, his observations are searing, and his book is a blessing'
  Kathryn Mannix, author of *With the End in Mind*

'This remarkable account of courage, fear and love will stay with you for a long time'   *Sun*

'An inspirational, ultimately heart-breaking account of experiencing life as the nervous system fails, shared with courage and humour'
Professor Stephen Westaby, author of *Fragile Lives*

A Short History
of Falling

Everything I Observed About
Love Whilst Dying

JOE HAMMOND

4th ESTATE • *London*

4th Estate
An imprint of HarperCollins*Publishers*
1 London Bridge Street
London SE1 9GF

www.4thEstate.co.uk

HarperCollins*Publishers*
1st Floor, Watermarque Building, Ringsend Road, Dublin 4, Ireland

First published in Great Britain in 2019 by 4th Estate
This 4th Estate paperback edition published in 2021

1

A catalogue record for this book is available from the British Library

ISBN 978-0-00-833994-4

The afterword was first published under the title
'I've been saying goodbye to my family for two years'
in the *Guardian* in December 2019.

Printed and bound in Great Britain by CPI Group (UK) Ltd, Croydon

MIX
Paper from
responsible sources
FSC™ C007454

This book is produced from independently certified FSC paper
to ensure responsible forest management

Find out more about HarperCollins and the environment at
www.harpercollins.co.uk/green

for Gill, Tom & Jimmy

Contents

Foreword xi

Tumbling 1
The Body 23
Doctor Tiago's Hydroelectric Power Plant 41
Cuckmere Haven 61
Losses 91
The Woman Who Lived in a Shoe 109
Gill 139
Mooto Nuney Disease 157
Fathers 177
What Dying Really Feels Like 209
Arrivals 235

Afterword 245
Acknowledgements 251

Foreword
by Gill Hammond

Things I have learnt about death
whilst living

How do you decide upon a day to die? For us, we had to find out when the doctors we needed were available; then we took note of the school holidays coming up, and finally we looked at the carer rota in place for that month. Who could we trust with Joe's death as much as we had trusted them with his life? It was a ludicrous situation really.

The next step was a meeting with the relevant doctors. What incredible women they were throughout this whole, surreal journey. They asked us, 'How did we imagine the process might unfold during which Joe would receive a huge amount of morphine to sedate him enough that his ventilator could be removed?' This was his wish – to withdraw from the treatment that had been keeping him alive these last six months. We were bemused. What were the options!? Apparently, some people choose to watch television and the programme of choice for their final breath of life is 'Countdown'. This gave Joe and me the giggles, and we said we thought we'd manage without any more conundrums than we had already.

How do you mark the days before the final day of your life? My top tip (in case you're interested) is to keep it simple. Our daily lives aren't fanfares and parades. In fact, the beauty of life is in all the tiny moments that are far more difficult to say goodbye to. The hand on a foot. The shared opinion on where the furniture should go. The stories of Tom and Jimmy's day. The excitement at seeing a woodpecker. A small fragment of the many moments before that final day.

Why am I sharing this with you? Well, that day arrived and it was the bravest thing I have ever witnessed. But it was also transformational in my understanding and acceptance of death. Death is coming to us all and I feel there is some new, unteachable knowledge to be gleaned from Joe's decision to allow it to come. To face it and know it. I think many people's understanding of death is no more nuanced than a Halloween-style dread. I know mine used to be. In fact, I don't know whether my younger self would even have wanted to pick up this book! And now? Now, I am relieved: sad, but no longer scared.

Why did Joe end his life? Well, it would have ended at some point and this disease wasn't going to give up. Other people may have chosen differently, but for Joe life had to have meaning and his increasing isolation from the world and particularly from the boys meant that he did not want to continue, and he wasn't afraid of dying.

I don't know where he is now and that is hard, but I do understand that nothing really dies and that matter just transforms into other forms. Tom and I have discussions about atoms and wonder whether daddy's atoms might just be dancing around us right now. No one knows for sure either way – so why not?

When I first met Joe he was wearing cords, a blazer, a leather satchel and of course, his black rimmed glasses. He looked like someone who should be on University Challenge but despite this, I was drawn to him. It wasn't love at first sight – it was curiosity and intrigue. To be honest, my immediate impression was that he might be interesting but he would be a bit wimpish, a bit wet – someone who wouldn't want to take a risk in life.

I can tell you, very specifically, the ways that led me to fall so much in love with Joe.

1   When, after only knowing me a few days, he walked across Oxford to come and light a fire for me in the flat where I was living because I couldn't get it started and there was a power cut.

2   When I watched him dive into the sea and fling himself with such abandon and joy from cliffs and off the edge of waterfalls.

3   When we strayed from our boring package holiday to navigate the heavily armed guards at the Egyptian/Israeli border just to see what could be found on the other side. This was two days before the hotel we ended up staying in was bombed.

4   When we stood at the stage door of the Royal Court stalking the actress Lindsay Duncan to give her a letter and a script. She replied later that night to say she must perform his monologue and she did!

5   When we roamed the frosty back streets of Paris for hours without a map or any idea of which way to get back to our coach. I was less impressed by Joe's determination to nurse some camembert cheese in his lap the whole 12-hour journey home, emitting frequent expressions of despair about its core temperature.

6   I fell more in love when I finally realised that I had to stop completing Joe's sentences because although Joe thought and spoke far slower than me, in reality, he said more with much less and his brain interpreted the world in such a unique and beautiful way.

7   Then came the day when he asked me 'What are you thinking?' I was perplexed. I wondered what I was supposed to say, but his manner and tone made me realise that he really wanted to *know* and he wanted me to tell him the truth. I don't know about you – but no one had really asked this of me before.

This simple question became so integral to our relationship. Something was created that became the foundation to everything in my life from that moment on. It was the simply complex notion of truth.

I knew that Joe would always tell me the truth and more importantly he would listen to my truths – even if they were hard to say or hard to hear. And this gave birth to something so precious and beautiful: trust.

For the very first time in my life, I knew exactly what love is. In my mind these two words united together as integrity. The huge presence of Joe was made more solid and substantial by his quest for truth and in the trust we found from sharing this. Joe lived by the Bettlheim quote: 'If you speak the truth then words come easily,' and what a beautiful craft he made with those words.

Joe always said that his work in schools for excluded, dysfunctional boys or in some of the most challenging care homes for young people was purely to finance writing. It's funny though, he kept ending up there. There are far easier ways to earn money! But in these places honesty and trust were at their most critical. Children, but especially those dispossessed, see things with such clarity and don't stand for the bullshit that most of us churn out. It gave Joe a perfect training ground for parenting, and anyone who saw him with his boys will know what power his solid presence has had upon them. I know this is embedded in their hearts and will bring them strength as they figure out the coming phases of their lives.

I'm aware that Joe might be starting to sound like a man of pure virtue, almost saint-like in his qualities. Of course, he was as flawed as all of us and we had our difficulties.

Tragic situations are, however, incredibly revealing – they illuminate our character, bring clarity and show us our most honest selves. I was in absolute awe of how Joe navigated this crazy disease. He sifted through his life to bring close the people and things that mattered most.

He let go of everything that didn't enrich our lives and he channeled his energy into sorting out his affairs, both the practical and the emotional. He never asked 'Why me?' and he told me there was no time to feel sorry for himself: such valuable lessons for living. He wanted to leave this world knowing that the boys and I were safe, and he made extraordinary things happen to achieve this. Humour and joy were part of everything – right until the very end.

So, I look back on our time together. And I remember Joe's face the day he returned from a 40-mile motorbike ride in Indonesia with six live crabs in his backpack. Or the pout on his face when he posed in the party wig that he would happily have worn every day. Or the pride we felt over a bucket full of mulberries he made us gather from Crystal Palace park with a step ladder on the day of the London riots. Or the joy at eating his homemade kimchi and the satisfaction he had seeing great vats of the stuff in our fridge. Or the wily way he would get his Nigerian friends to cook him Jollof rice by stoking rivalry between them! But it was with Tom and Jimmy where you saw the soul of Joe at work. Nothing mattered more to him than his two boys and he was – without exaggeration – an inspirational father.

I was privileged to hold his hand to the very end. I kissed him as he took his final breaths. I witnessed his bravery and spirit and I hope I can continue to find this strength within me. I am grateful for the time we have had. I am grateful for our cheeky, charming children. I am grateful for the food he cooked and the curious things that would make him laugh. I am grateful for his huge arms and loving embrace. I am grateful for all the things we taught each other and the integrity that glued us together and I am incredibly grateful for all the adventures, both the whacky and the tough. He would actually have been useless on University Challenge.

My grief is eased knowing that Joe is to be found amongst my friends but also with you, the reader, who will take this little journey into your lives. And I am comforted to know that at the end, it really is okay.

Tumbling

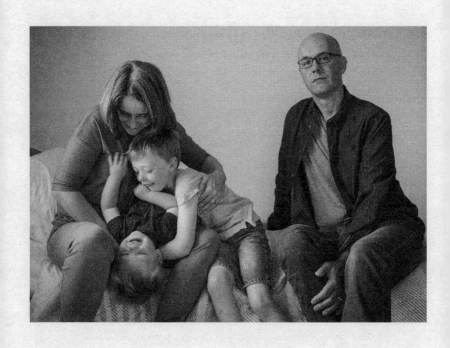

If I could just stop falling over, this would be a funnier book. I'm a big man and I'm starting to cause a lot of damage. I've just written off a kitchen cabinet, and two weeks ago I dislocated my shoulder on the bedroom floor. Quite recently I fell into my son's empty cot, but that was a peaceful experience. The sides of the cot snapped inwards, swaddling me in very fine, soft, white mesh. Given how unsafe I am at the moment, this felt OK. I decided to remain there, looking around. It was quiet. It would have been nice to sleep, but then my other son – my six-year-old – walked in.

If I'm near other people and I sway this way or that, it can seem balletic – like one of those trust games when a person is encouraged to tuck their arms inwards and let others prevent their fall. But often I find myself alone or out of reach, and from a height of six foot three falling always takes so *long*. Or it feels like it. I seem to have plenty of time to think and notice and worry in that quiet moment before impact. And that's been quite frightening. Just observing the slowness of my descent and picking both a landing spot and part of my body that seems most capable of taking the impact. And whenever I hit the floor, or something on the way down to the floor, it's never a funny thing or a funny moment. Never something funny that I want to write about the next day. Last week I fell and split my head open in the shower. And I just lay there. Because if I fall, I can't use my arms to get back up. I lay there, beached and soapy on the white-tiled floor, with the water raining down turning pale pink around me. And my wife running in like a Greenpeace activist to a seal cull.

I'm getting to the point when I shall look back on these falls as moments of luxury. From a wheelchair or a hoist or a hospital bed, I'll view these early days of motor neurone disease as a time of freedom. A time when toppling or tripping or tumbling was actually possible. Because I can put my finger through the place where muscles used to be in my legs, right through to the tendons, and can feel something like the substructure of myself emerging. And it's not a particularly good sign, but it's not everything. It's just the physical body. This book is everything – the experience of my body as it changes and declines. The experience of saying goodbye to those I love. I'm scared – I know I am. But it feels strangely OK. And surprising too. I'm going to tell you about it. The story of my end, or as close as I can get to it.

*

The first I knew was about fifteen months ago. It was the sensation that I had a fresh piece of chewing gum stuck to the sole of my foot. Feet feel bigger when they don't lift properly. My big clown foot, and the funny slapping sound as I ran for a bus. And perhaps I could have fixed this by attaching a piece of string to my big right toe. But where do you stop with such things? How much of a marionette can one person be?

I was walking like a passenger in the aisle of a plane going through gentle turbulence. It's the walk someone would make just prior to the seat-belt lights coming back on again – that medium level of mid-flight turbulence. But not on a plane: on the ground. On the way to make a sandwich or brush my teeth. Just walking. With my palms face down, as if steadying myself on the headrests of non-existent passengers.

My first fall was when I was walking Tom to school. We had joined with several mums and their children and it was a cheerful occasion. I made my way to the edge of the pavement to widen our group so that I could chat alongside what was now a phalanx of mums. But as I put my right foot down, I felt only the very edge of the kerb. I'd expected more underfoot. And the rest of my foot fell away from the group. Not off the edge of a cliff, off the edge of a kerb, but somehow I kept falling. There was no correction from either leg, as if each were too polite to be the first to move. So the whole structure of me went down. It all landed between two parked cars. About five or six children looked over me, including Tom, and a number of the mums. Something about the choreography perplexed – I think we all felt that. After the briefest of moments, most of us started laughing. And then I got up and we laughed some more. We laughed about it again when our walks next coincided.

But Tom laughed the least. He wasn't particularly upset; he just didn't find it funny. He's logged quite a few falls since then. Several weeks ago he was with a friend as she listened to an account of her aunt's recent fall and then remarked that adults don't do such things. My son corrected her immediately. It was a factually incorrect statement, and he is good at spotting those.

*

I next fell while trying to do an impression of a pop-up toaster. This was some months later. Actually, there had been other falls in the intervening period, but nothing calamitous. Nothing I remember. By this time we were living in Portugal, where the tiled floors are so shiny that I can't think of anywhere less suitable for a man with my predisposition towards falling. And this was just part of the adventure. A new life on shiny floors. On this occasion I fell and slammed the back of my head against a radiator. Tom and Jimmy, who was then just over a year old, were sitting on Tom's bed wrapped in towels after an evening bath. Tom had just correctly identified my washing machine and there had been other white goods, as well as a vacuum cleaner. With the toaster, I keeled over because my left leg achieved the elevation my right one couldn't. It was a buckled-cartwheel move, and when my head made impact it was the deep vibrating sound from the pipes that shocked us all. I lay back with my head wedged uncomfortably forwards against the steel pillow. After a few moments, Jimmy started crying; then Tom. I looked over at them. Their tears. Their crumpled faces. And a nasally sound like two interlinked air-raid sirens being squeezed out through their ears.

There's so much more indignity in failed silliness. The thought of no longer being the clown brings me as close as anything to feeling defeated. A lot rests on being able to impersonate a toaster. I don't think I've ever wanted to spend more than five minutes with anyone who isn't in some way capable of being a clown. And my feelings of loss are at their most profound when these opportunities evade me. If I can't brush my teeth in the style of a camel. Or getting dressed in the mornings and no longer being able to chuck my discarded pyjamas at my children.

I've noticed that nothing can trigger tearfulness quite like an unexpected sound. This was the case with my toaster and the deep clang of the radiator, but also with the time I wrote off the kitchen cutlery drawer. I'd grown weaker, but was reluctant to give up my role as house cook. In the kitchen I needed to hold on to the counter to keep myself upright. So it was all quite sloppy; a little desperate. I'd chop an onion by throwing a knife at it or chuck a used spoon at the sink from twenty feet away. On this occasion my energy was particularly low. We had guests and I should have asked for help. I remember I didn't bother counting the cutlery. I just shovelled it up and left the drawer open, then spun around towards the dining table. I shouldn't have been spinning. I shouldn't have been manoeuvring in such a casual way. But I doled out the correct cutlery at the table and spun back towards the drawer with the spares, catching the left toe of my rubber trainers on the shiny tiled floor and my right spastic foot on the heel of my static left ankle. Having reached tipping point, there wasn't a chance my legs could save me. By this stage of the disease, rather than legs, my upper body was being supported by a creaky twin-set of large Victorian steel stanchions. I knew I was falling. It's passive knowledge. Knowing it's about to happen; knowing I can't prevent it. In a cartoon, I would be whistling at this point, or checking a wristwatch. But actually, in that moment, I was gauging my total 'arms outstretched' length, my distance to the cutlery tray, the fixed position of my feet, and had calculated that my hands would become parallel with the cutlery tray at the point at which my falling body would reach an angle of thirty-five degrees from the floor. And I had judged it well: that's exactly where my hands were. But I had not allowed for the velocity with which my hands would be travelling through the air, and this was considerable. My upper limbs crashed through the open drawer before I could reasonably subdivide into forks, knives and spoons, bringing the drawer and its contents down with me, in much the same way that simulated films show the collision of an asteroid into Earth, bringing an end to the age of dinosaurs.

*

My role as house cook began sixteen years ago. I'd known Gill a week, so we weren't even living together by this point. I was lingering outside her kitchen, trying to catch sight of her as she prepared a meal. I didn't know what to do and I was a little nervous. A little expectant. I heard clattering sounds and moved to take up a better vantage point. I remember the excitement of then seeing Gill through the frame of the doorway. She was holding a tin of tuna, trying to get the contents out. She was thrusting it downwards, the way a person might try to get some very stiff ketchup from a bottle, the way someone would do this when they don't know the technique of slapping the base of the bottle with the palm of the hand. She was trying so hard. And I have always remembered the repetitions of the despairing downward plunge of her arm. That repeated, forlorn, hopeless, futile, beguiling, beautiful movement of her arm through the air.

*

It's hard to live the losses moment to moment, accepting them as they arise, dispensing with pieces of the self fluently like a bag of birdseed strewn into a flock of pigeons. Lying on my back on the shiny tiled floor, I was struck by the amount of metal and detritus that can be loaded into one cutlery drawer. I was turning as I hit the drawer, so my hands and wrists connected side-on to the open drawer and the impact turned me completely. I couldn't necessarily see what was lying all around me, but the sound of falling metal seemed to continue like hail on a skylight. And I lay, arms outstretched, on this sea of steel and crud. A friend and her sister were staying with us, and each got up and took my arms, raising me to a marginally more dignified seated position. Directly in front of me were Tom and Jimmy, standing side by side. Three foot tall and two foot tall. Their lips were beginning to agitate, like four pink caterpillars rippling across a leaf. Sitting on my bum amidst the debris, I watched as their faces crumpled and they again began squeezing air-raid sirens out through their ears. Once they had levered me up, the two sisters began gathering in all the items. It was a job I desperately wanted. I wanted to be down there, on my knees. Putting it all back together again. The spoons in one place, the forks, the knives. The masher, the crusher, the bashers, the smashers. The togs, the bottle tops, the skewers, the openers. And then a dustpan and brush for all the accumulated dust and dirt.

*

From an early age I dreamt of falling. For many years, this simple dream included nothing more than a matchstick or a marble or something small like that. It was just me and these little bits and pieces suspended in space. It was something like the very beautiful children's television programme from the 1980s called *Button Moon*, which told the story of Mr Spoon and his friends in a bits and pieces universe. My own version wasn't quite as charming. There was no ground or environment – just these items – and in the dream I would be concentrating on these little things. My hands were there and in this dream my job existed to make sure nothing fell. And this really was the crux of it – that nothing must fall. Because if it did, everything would end.

I used to listen to my parents fighting at night. It was dark outside. And if you're an older child, you turn your music up, or you open your door and shout down the stairs, slamming the door back shut behind you. But if you're young – or very young – nothing seems separate from who you are. Sounds settle on the skin and are then absorbed, as if they are your own, as if these problems are your own.

I had this dream in largely the same form, for many years. Always the same task – to keep the world in place. I think the pressure was something like a bomb-disposal expert might feel if they were somehow forced to experience their job as a child. And, of course, within this dream something would always fall and I would wake with the certain knowledge that not a bit of the world remained.

*

As my legs began to weaken, and my right spastic leg began to stiffen, I was excited to find that I could improve my balance by walking around with a book on my head. Tom had a Paddington Bear book that worked best. It was hard and heavy and square and I seemed more conscious of my movement with this book. Less likely to fall. It was the story of Paddington's journey from Darkest Peru, his arrival at Paddington station, and his early home life with Mr and Mrs Brown. I made this discovery about a month or so following my diagnosis. At around this time my arms began a spontaneous adaptation to the heaviness in my legs. I widened my gait and began purposefully reaching out with my arms, and breathing out with each movement. It was loosely inspired by a session or two of t'ai chi that I once did, but it felt like my creation. Or an evolution, perhaps, towards life as an anthropod.

I cherished this time. I felt more aware of my body than at any other time in my life. I wanted to feel my body and be in my body because I knew I was losing it. I think about this time and often wonder what would have developed had I not caught a leg on the strap of a bag I'd left on the bedroom floor. Part of me wishes I'd decided to make impact with my face, not my shoulder, because I later decided that the disablement of my shoulder accelerated certain aspects of this disease. But

I think all this fall did was to create a kink in the line of my body's development. The perception of acceleration, maybe some actual acceleration, but not much. The abrupt end to this fertile period helped me to mythologize my short life as an insect. That's all.

Because the truth is that I was actually declining through this period. I just enjoyed the thought that I wasn't. I think the fall ended one kind of hope, but it didn't end all kinds of hope. The creative life gets harder and darker and more real. But life is not worse than it was before. It doesn't have less value. It's not less interesting. Not at all. As I get weaker, less a part of this world, or less a part of what I love, less a part of my family's life, I can perceive its edges with fantastic clarity. I can lie against it, lolling my arm over the edge, running my fingers around the rim. And this is where I am.

*

I might now notice that I haven't fallen for a while, rather than that I have fallen. This normalization is just taking shape. I had one of these quotidian falls last week. As I was heading out of the kitchen, I caught my sandal in the indentation of the grouting between the floor tiles. My wrists were attached to crutches so that, falling through the door, my body and both arms behaved like three portly figures bustling to be the first out. I was aware of a lot of jostling between these separate components of my body. The momentum took my torso through ahead of the other two fat fellows, with my arms pinned back behind as they followed. As these three oafs who comprised my body clattered through the doorway, what landed first was my chin. And because of the order of my body, my shoulders splayed out and my palms landed with a splat on either side. One crutch was still painfully attached to my wrist, cuffing me to the ground. And my body transmitted to me the physical impression that I had been pinned to the floor by an arresting officer. I didn't initially attempt to move. I wasn't particularly hurt; it was more the feeling of profound dismay at having to work out a way to get up from the floor.

Having previously described the siren sounds of my children after they witnessed one of my falls, this fall provided further evidence of the transition along the scale from horror to tedium. There was a brief sound of upset being squeezed out through Jimmy's ears, but nothing like the previous episodes and nothing from Tom. They had seen it all before. Daddy had now been seen on the floor on a number of occasions, so the sound on this occasion was something like that brief attention-seeking pulse from a police siren that makes you wonder why they bothered. I think Jimmy soon thought better of it and he continued emptying the recycling out from its various containers. Gill came to help, but I told her I was OK for the moment and, dribbling into the carpet, suggested she finish grilling the fish fingers. Tom stepped over me on his way up the stairs. I could hear supper being plated up and I wanted to stay put – perhaps for ever. I was seriously considering the possibility. And nothing about that thought felt in any way abnormal.

*

I now spend a lot of time in my pants and people come and go. It's getting harder to put my clothes on and the heating here is quite good. As I write this, I'm in my pants, and I'm looking down at my T-shirt which displays the remains of two splodges of the beetroot and squash soup I had for lunch. A lot of me is not as decorous as it once was and it's in this unvarnished state that I now tend to find myself, groaning on the floor, after the latest fall.

Having fallen, it's now impossible for me to get myself back up. That's been the case for months, but now Gill and I can't quite manage it together. The most recent example resulted in quite a lot of pain and the unfortunate reprisal of my recently healed rotator-cuff injury. On this occasion, Gill was the first to arrive and

I was able to roll over on to my back to have the usual conversation about whether I was or wasn't OK. I spent a minute or two being aware of the furrows on Gill's brow, but then Jimmy swung in through the door. He was smiling broadly and, having not actually seen me fall, appeared simply tickled by the experience of looking down at me.

A visiting friend of ours was the last to arrive. I suppose I mention all this because, with this particular episode, I'm partly writing about dignity and how I just don't bother with it any more. Attending to my dignity would take too long and would consume a vast amount of Gill's time. Behind every sponged and smartly dressed disabled person has to be someone else's considerable and uncredited commitment.

It took us a few minutes, but the mechanics of raising me up were extremely effective. I'm no engineer so I cannot explain the considerable biomechanical benefit of a single hand placed lightly under my bottom. Under normal conditions I struggle to raise myself from a chair but, with a hand inserted just under my bum, exerting marginal upward pressure, I seem to experience very little upward difficulty. On this occasion we were trying to raise me up from the floor but with the compensation of six hands. I found it particularly affecting that two of them belonged to Jimmy – the boy I should be cradling

in my big Daddy arms. My wife, my son, a friend –
all managing with my near dead weight. I could never
previously have conceived of six hands seeking upward
traction from my bottom. But the operation worked. In
yesterday's pants and a dirty T-shirt, I'd made it to sitting – on the edge of the bed – relieved and looking out
at my trio of helpers.

*

For almost six months we'd been living on the side of
a mountain in rural central Portugal, and then I was
diagnosed and we fell all the way down to the bottom.
We fell through the pines and the eucalyptus, bump-
ing and clattering against the trunks, brushing through
the foliage. We cartwheeled and bounced and slipped
– an eighteen-month-old baby, a six-year-old boy and a
mum and dad. And it was remarkable that we fell a mile
downwards from high up on the mountainside, with the
speed of falling objects, but sustained no external injur-
ies – no cuts or grazes. Nothing visible. Everything that
hurt was on the inside – the disappointment and the
shock and the sadness.

It had been Gill's idea to come to Portugal. She had
been on maternity leave with Jimmy and dreamt up the
idea, and we carried through with it. Our flat had been
rented out and we were experimenting with a different

kind of living. Tom had not enjoyed his start to school life in the UK but now found himself in a tiny bilingual school surrounded by cherry trees, where he spent half his day constructing shelters from old tractor tyres and mud and fallen masonry and discarded timber.

And Gill and I spent our days together in the sun, learning a new language and eating the oranges and cabbages and potatoes that neighbours would leave on our doorstep. And I don't know how long this life would have gone on for, but I do know, if my diagnosis had been for something sweeter, something fixable, that our journey home to the UK would have been slower – not off the side of a precipice, with the rocks, the stones and the blood-red earth flashing by.

*

I had a moment yesterday when my fingers went reaching for the finial on the banister at the first landing. I looked at my fingers. They were playing a little piano melody in the air. I could feel the slightest sense that my body had moved backwards, rather than forwards. That my hand was doing the opposite of reaching; it was withdrawing. And that this worried me. It was only a faint sensation at this point. The very gentle transitive feeling that a treetop must feel just after the axe has finished its work on the trunk. A subtle movement at first but with full knowledge of the carnage that will follow. It's the worst kind of terror, the one that begins with such gentility. Knowing what it means; what it would mean for my body. The steepness of the gradient behind me and the hardness of its edges. The damage I would do to my limbs if I were to fall back in that moment. Falling back and needing to take it. The quiet minutes and hours and years of the falling moment. And the thoughts of my wife as she would come running. What all this would mean. Of lives disturbed. By a set of fingers flailing short.

This is a special subcategory of falls – perhaps the worst kind – because they linger and they haunt, they spill and they drift. These are the almost falls – the ones that never happen; the ones that nearly happen. The moment of knowing a fall is happening. Not fearing it. *Knowing* it. Even if that moment is fractional, and then snapping out of that space. It's the waterboarding equivalent of falling, because it feels like it's happening but it's not. The heart turns inside out like a rubber cup and then pings back into shape. It's time travel, or two parallel moments coexisting: the disastrous one and the banal one, with thoughts rattling helplessly between them like a pebble in a bucket. The finial was out of reach, but the banister rails weren't. I never forget the almost falls. Not the bad ones.

One pebble has been rattling around for the last nine years, getting more clattery with each recollection. I was on a path on the edge of a ravine. I must have stopped for something. A view? Maybe I needed a piss. Gill was ahead. I could see her disappearing as she traversed the sharp cliff along a loose, flinty path. We were trekking on the Indian side of the Himalayas, without a guide. We were alone. And as I skipped forward to catch up, my toe caught a rock and my two insteps collided. After a stumble forwards, the thick sole of my right boot skidded flat and I came to a stop. I was on my own in the silence. Gill was out of view, with the precipice just ahead. I thought of the degrees by which falls can happen: the strength or slightness of the connection that one toecap might make with one heel, in the process of stumbling and clattering. And how close I came to a more prolonged stumble, and then to nothing, to disappearing over the edge, in the silence, out of view. Imagining the experience of Gill as she stepped back on herself into a mystery. To an empty path. It's the silence of that moment that concentrates this memory. The fitting stage that it was for an ending. The intimation of an ending, even though it wasn't.

Every thought I have had about that moment has been more profound than the one I had at the time. I shook it off, but it has stayed with me and has grown in the dark with each recollection. I didn't mention it to Gill when it happened. I just trotted on and caught up. Because nothing actually happened – nothing that I felt I could communicate.

I'm falling now. But this time it is real. Unlike you, perhaps, I *know* I am dying. And because of that I fear it less.

The Body

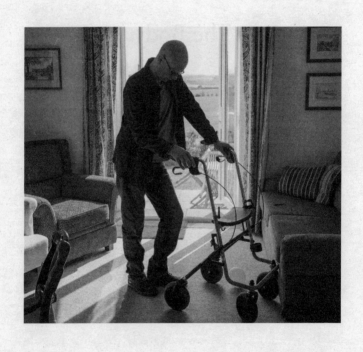

As I progress down the upstairs landing, holding on to my four-wheel disability rollator, I invariably glance through the open door of the bathroom. It's become a pattern. Glancing through the door at the metallic frame that holds my raised plastic disability toilet seat. This momentary experience reminds me of the times in my life when I've walked past specialist disability shops, gazing absently at all the unlikely paraphernalia from other people's lives. This world of experience in one shop. And this is what it feels like, seeing this con-traption installed around my toilet. It's other people's lives; not my own. But each time I remember that it is mine, and that's quite shocking.

I think I feel the same level of original shock on every occasion. And these are largely the same feelings that I have about every disability item I own: the cone-shaped device for putting on my socks, the grabbing and reaching implements, the rails, the splint, the stroller,

Dr Seuss's fantastical self-washing wires and brushes. New items arrive almost daily and I am unexpectedly becoming the curator of the Museum of my own Decline. How did this happen? Because it wasn't so long ago that I was walking past these shops. I was on the pavement looking in. And now I am inside.

*

If you're disabled, London beggars don't ask you for money. They don't even make eye contact. I discovered this whilst visiting the UK at Christmas, travelling through London on my own. This was a few months before we had to move back permanently, and I was being disabled all by myself. I must have seemed quite unsteady because it was my first experience as the recipient of help from strangers. I found this exciting. I don't feel excitement any more. But at that time it was exhilarating in the way that all transportive experiences can be exhilarating. Like an acting student with a begging bowl or a celebrity in a fat suit. Except that it was me. The most complete version of me that I would ever be.

I changed trains at East Croydon and deliberately trailed a woman with a crutch who had a spastic leg like mine. I sat quite near her but realized she was much younger, with MS. Then I felt like an older man stalking a younger woman, which I briefly was. I gravitate towards people with a bad leg like me. At Three Bridges station there was a man of about my age with an even slower walk than me. He was dressed smartly and clearly trying to sustain some kind of job. I was coming from the other direction and had enough time to become excited by the way his leg was swaying wildly – just like mine. It was rush hour. Not an easy time to be thrashing your leg around. I wanted to wave or to say something; or communicate to my brother with an upward turn of my eyebrows. And because we were heading in opposite directions I knew our unacknowledged time together would be fleeting. He needed help, from crutches at least, but he had nothing. I was impressed by his lack of speed. I should have been going a little slower. Or I should have stopped to think, but I ended up doing the opposite. I picked up speed and felt momentarily jaunty. It's what I must have wanted. I was racing along. And that was it; the moment for connection was gone.

He's not the first person I've picked out, wondering whether he or she is the same as me. Wanting to ask. I fabricated a notion that this man's symptoms might have been further on than mine. Perhaps he had been slow to refer himself, and was soldiering on. A man who was continuing to work in the face of considerable difficulty – wondering why his foot wouldn't lift off the ground. Wondering why he was always toppling over like an old wet tree in the rain. And waiting for it all to stop, for the body to return, to heal, because that is what the body does.

I don't think I'm looking for my comrades any more. Not with quite that expectation. Or with that sense of shocking newness I want to share. But still, when I'm with a friendly physio or occupational therapist, I often end up asking about their other patients. I must want to find someone like me. Someone out there with children who is where I am with this disease. Someone out there who is writing about it. Wanting it to be OK. Willing it to be OK. I want to meet this person.

*

It's shocking to me that I have a spastic leg. I'm struck by its arcing trajectory, its banana-shaped inefficiency, and by the sticks I use to compensate for it. And by the wheelchair I will one day be consigned to, the toileting aids that await me, disfigurement, the premature ageing. These are all shocking to me; I'm calm about it, but still shocked. I'm calmly shocked.

All my life I've convinced myself that I have a remarkably striking physical appearance. Unfortunately, I have been capable of believing that almost anything about me, or almost anything I've done, might be remarkably brilliant. I have been afflicted by this delusion for my entire life. There's nothing unusual about this. It's just the dreariness of narcissism. Only the route towards narcissism is unique. The real stuff. The narcissism itself, the affliction, is dull, boring and predictable. And as with all narcissism, mine has an obverse side which is equally true and equally present: the unrelenting conviction that when I'm not being remarkably clever and beautiful, I'm being remarkably stupid and ugly.

But now I'm living with a concept that is neither. It's not life at the end of either of these two extremes. It's not even on the same linear scale. These days I'm preoccupied by the surprises in my life. The way the body reminds me of myself. The saliva I'm now collecting in my mouth. It's this. It's all the tiny signals I experience. The not swallowing. The lagoons beneath my tongue. These pools of saliva don't interest the narcissist in me. In the presence of such novel details I've finally found a way to bore him. With my actual body. The volumes of swallowed juices that sluice away like the downpipe from a toilet stack. Sometimes when I inhale they inadvertently skim backwards with a splutter and a choke. Or, if I'm lying on my front, a small amount disappears over the curve of my bottom lip. Just a little for now, over the side of the bed. Just a tiny stream from a toy teapot. A darkened dot on the carpet. Everything starts as something small. There are no shocks. This is a gentle kind of devastation.

When I was a much younger man I spent a year or so not being narcissistic. I had found God, briefly. I knew him for a year. He loved me and I loved him and my narcissism ebbed away. I felt the tension in my body release. I felt my 25-year-old body open up, after many years of tightness. When I no longer felt I knew him, my narcissism returned. My body closed again, as if a season had passed. This sounds glib, but it's the truth. And even though I lost hold of what I had found, I don't think a person ever completely loses what they have had. I'd lived with a level of shock and confusion my entire life, but something had been lifted that was never completely pushed back down again.

And now, being a man with a spastic leg, finding myself being wheeled through an airport in a wheelchair, as I was earlier today, I realize this is the culmination. It's finishing something, finally and decisively. I'm a man with a disability. My body is the truth now and it's saving me from myself. I have all these losses, and feel a kind of freedom in that. With each awkward, spasmodic movement, or the difficulty I have wiping my own bottom, or with the slur developing in my voice, the narcissist recedes. There's nothing for him here. Not any more. It's death to him. The phoney.

You wasted a lot of my life. Nothing you did was ever real.

*

In the weeks and months that followed my diagnosis I received dozens of suggestions about how I might combat my decline. Some fell into the category of *tonic* and these included several exotic examples, such as a paste made from mixing water with powdered scrapings from reindeer-horn velvet. I was also advised to start my day with warming spices, so that I might have a ginger or a cinnamon tea. Or I could have eggs for breakfast and cook them with turmeric and cumin.

Other suggestions have been less to do with ingestion than the functions or processes that I could add or alter within my body. In one of the loveliest examples a friend espoused the medical benefits that singing could offer me. A more prosaic example was that I could slow the progression of the disease by chewing my food more slowly.

In some cases, these suggestions have been delivered with little confidence. Perhaps they're offered if a person feels awkward and wants to think of something positive to say – so that it might be something they'd heard about from someone or caught as a snippet on the radio. On one occasion I received a text from a friend to inform me that a new drugs trial in India had yielded miraculous results. I texted back to ask for more details but, unfortunately, he was unable to be more specific. I wondered if he might have the name of a town or medical institution so that I could narrow it down a little but, no, it was just something that was happening broadly within the nation of India.

Others have been far more confident in their approaches – strikingly so. I'm particularly thinking of two parents from Tom's previous school in Portugal. In both cases, I didn't know the people involved that well and they had first learnt of my condition from chatting to another parent in the playground. In the case of these two women it was interesting to note some common attributes to their communication style. Both times the initial engagement involved gently touching my elbow and very sensitively, very earnestly, leading me away from a mingled group of parents. What I then noticed was the closeness of the physical space they occupied, so that the intensity of the eye contact lent the exchange a certain gravity and seriousness.

As for the suggestions themselves, they were both to do with diet. I have noticed that people can be at their most fervent when making claims that this or that diet can combat my decline. I group these two approaches together because each person espoused a dietary regime which, as far as I can tell, appeared to be the diametric opposite of the other. So that one of them was suggesting a diet based exclusively on fats and animal protein, whilst the other suggested a vegetarian diet of brown rice, sea vegetables and pulses.

As these two separate discussions continued, and the volume of parents surrounding us thinned significantly, it became clear that these two women weren't actually prescribing a bespoke cure for my specific neurological condition; in fact, it wasn't entirely clear that they knew what my condition was. It didn't appear to be the case that the diets could specifically prevent my motor neurones dying. Instead I was offered the reassurance that they themselves, and their family – as notably healthy and flourishing individuals – were also following this dietary regime and that anyone else in their right mind should be doing the same. As time went on, and we met repeatedly in the playground – and it became clear that I wasn't following their guidance – the looks on their faces conveyed a saintly form of disappointment. I had been offered *the way* but clearly lacked piety. In this respect, it seemed that I hadn't been approached by two friendly and knowledgeable parents but by two variants of the same religion.

The list of cures I receive continues to grow. It seems important for some people to feel that they can do something about what's happening to me. Sometimes this is offered in a caring or despairing way and sometimes it's evangelical. But in all cases it feels like a frustration with the idea that things *happen*: the idea that we all might grow old or that any of us might contract an illness or a disease and not be able to do anything about it, or the idea that none of us really possess control over our lives. For many people this is clearly unbearable and intolerable, so that just *being* is frightening – and that the only possible sane response is to be *doing* something.

*

The loss of motor neurones begins with a display – something visible just beneath the surface of the skin. You could watch my wrist and observe tiny pulsing movements working their way up my arm – like a trapped cricket trying to find its way out. Or if you were to place an open hand on the side of my neck, you might wait there for a moment and then suddenly squeak or let out a little 'Ooh!' as you snatch your hand away.

These are the flickerings of a light bulb before the plink and fizz of a blown filament. Tiny faltering premonitions of loss – a kind of panic or disturbance in a muscle that is losing its sense of purpose within the body. For some reason, these twitches make me think of earthworms after the rain – when the soil is claggy and they come to the surface for oxygen: the way they blindly pop out of the soil, flailing and wriggling in the unnatural habitat of the air.

When I hold Gill's hand the sensation transmits through the ends of my fingers or through the muscle at the base of my thumb. It's hard to feel her flinching from the movements of my body – from the subcutaneous crickets and the earthworms popping up for air. Hard to reassure her that at least the fibres are still looking for connection – that they haven't given up – that it's not the end.

But these fasciculations are beginning to get less frequent now – like that moment at the end of a garden fireworks display when the nostrils are pleasingly filled with sulphur and the last firework in the box fizzles out and someone hands you a sausage roll, and you're standing by the embers of the bonfire watching the ghost of an image from a burnt-out sparkler.

*

A couple of times in the writing of this book I've discarded more extended metaphors that attempted to convey what this disease is – and its effect on the body. In the first, I was describing a steel suspension bridge: the way the bridge appears to function normally, whilst up above, and out of view of the traffic, the cables supporting the stanchions are snapping one by one. Over time, fewer of the cables are taking more of the strain until, finally, a steel stanchion begins to creak and wobble. From this point, decay continues much as it did before but now visible and obvious.

The second of my abandoned metaphors employed the image of a corner shop, in which shelf items mysteriously disappear through the walls or the floor. Increasingly, the stock appears sporadic and the shop becomes less useful as a place for anyone to reliably buy their groceries. Sometimes the shop door opens and the visitor looks around, having arrived here through habit, forgetting that the place has fallen into decline. Others still choose to come, if they have the time, remembering what it was – or they maintain their shopping habit out of nostalgia and affection.

It's so easy to reach for these metaphors of loss and decay, and I think this has something to do with the absence of concrete information about what this disease actually is, or what causes it. No one appears to know why or how or when motor neurones die within the body; why the line of communication between brain and muscular tissue breaks down. It remains a mystery, so that in thinking and writing about my degenerating body, imagery and imagination can be everything. This is the reason why, despite writing about the removal of extended metaphors, I'm nonetheless tripping over smaller, rat-size examples of imagery darting in from every angle.

But when reaching too far into metaphor, the experience of what something *actually* feels like becomes lost – and because I feel this experience so profoundly within my body, it's description that really matters to me. I've had my moment here – descending into metaphor – to help explain the little I know about how this disease works. But I don't experience the disease, I experience my body, and this is what interests me. I know enough not to think that sea vegetables or reindeer velvet can delay its course. Of course, somewhere out there, a reason exists for why these neurones die, and there's probably something out there that will stop this. Maybe it *is* sea vegetables! But these dart-throwing investigations can't be anything to do with me – not whilst the shamans are still shaking their sticks at the moon. They don't interest me.

All that interests me is being with people – and with my body as it dies – and writing about it.

*

On the other side of the room Tom and Jimmy are flapping on our bed like unnetted herrings on the deck of a trawler. Gill's laughing and the boys are squealing, but

I'm over here with my recliner all the way back resting my tongue on the floor of my mouth. It's unusual to be this much on the outside of an escapade, not even to be enjoying the fact that my children are so happy. I could be in an adjacent hotel room or in a split time frame. There are other moments when I will sit and enjoy: laughing or smiling at acrobatics, or boofing a pillow into someone's face. But on this occasion my recliner is tilted back and I'm interested in the difference between the roofs of the two terraced houses I can see through the window. The slate on one roof is clean and new, but where the roof becomes another property the roofer has left the moss-barnacled slates unchanged. It's the same roof. A shared roof. But the two parts are cared for as if they exist in different continents.

Gill and I can still talk and talk when we get the chance, and I can still read books to the boys, but this evening my facial and tongue muscles have grown more tired than usual. I spent the day on the phone to estate agents, solicitors and various health professionals. I became hoarse quite early on in the day and then the susceptible muscle at the base of my tongue began to ache. I used my reserves and now I'm spent. So I've tilted myself back in this moment and taken myself away. To a time, perhaps a year from now, when the voice is gone and the face is gone. And my hands can no longer make signs. Preparing for disability is like going on holiday somewhere new and wondering what clothes to pack. For now, I'm scouting it out. Just temporarily – just for an hour or two. Being elsewhere, in an expanding private world; a world I will get to know. I'm glad to feel it first. Preparing for when I will be looking out at the life of my family. Knowing that I was out there once. The clown. The protagonist. The herring.

Doctor Tiago's Hydroelectric Power Plant

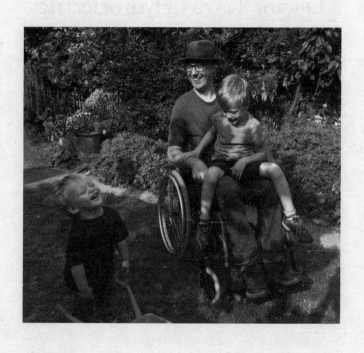

In the moments before Doctor Tiago called me in, I was propping up a wall with my shoulder. When you spend a lot of time in hospitals being undiagnosed, you start propping up walls and lounging about and picking your nose in waiting rooms. And not being prepared for certainty when it comes.

An hour or two before, Doctor Tiago had been scratching away at my body with a pin. But before all this, I'd been lying on my front and waiting. I could hear him scrabbling about, trying to find something. I heard the clasp of his bag. I heard him stirring the contents around. The thin metallic sound of a cabinet door being opened and shut. A drawer sliding open and then slamming shut. He'd been searching in the room for something sharp. I realized that later. I don't know where he got the pin from. Thinking about it, I was lying face down: it might not have been a pin. What was it? This wasn't the first time he'd taken to me with something sharp. He'd made some preliminary etchings on my last visit, but this time he was dragging the pin rapidly across and around my back and legs in wide swirling motions; an impressionist holding their brush at the very tip of the handle, standing back from their canvas and operating in broad strokes. He'd stop for a moment and then start again. Then he'd have another thought and drag the pin wildly in a different direction. And when I sat up he was holding his chin and thinking.

'Your face is lopsided.'

'Is it?'

I really like Doctor Tiago. His smile is perhaps the broadest and most expressive smile I have ever encountered. It is so broad and all-encompassing that it seems to subsume his entire face, right up to his eyebrows. A couple of months earlier he had found me wandering the corridors, having arrived at the hospital for a non-existent appointment. He seemed much more like a very young and enthusiastic uncle than a doctor. On that occasion he set up an impromptu clinic in what seemed like a stationery cupboard and we went from there. In all my time with the hospital, I was never really aware of how appointments happened. They just did. It was all quite miraculous. And so I don't mind that he put so much effort into trying to find a brain tumour. He was clearly misled by my face. Even the neurologist who did my CAT scan said I had a brain tumour. They couldn't find any evidence of a tumour. This didn't matter. They remained convinced. Cheerfully so. Apparently a brain tumour is great news.

I wonder why it is important to know. It always seems so very important, particularly for doctors. But surely they seldom know. Or they seldom *really* know. Doctor Tiago 'knew' I had a brain tumour within five minutes of meeting me. But this wasn't knowing; this was confidence. We'd have had a better conversation without confidence getting in the way. There's so much to simply not know about the body. I'd prefer a person who really knows about something (like Doctor Tiago) to tell me all the myriad fascinating things they don't know. Because however much a person knows about something, that *knowing* is minuscule compared to what they don't know. A scale demonstration of this would involve standing next to a mountain and pouring a kilo bag of sugar on the ground. Standing back and comparing these two mounds would give the onlooker a visual comparison between the little that is known about anything by anyone (the sugar) and the vastness of what is unknown about everything by everyone (the mountain). None of us know. Even the most knowledgeable amongst us don't know. Doctor Tiago didn't know. I'd like to have spent more time with Doctor Tiago not knowing.

This was the third time I had seen Doctor Tiago. Each time he would make me clench my teeth and then he'd nod with certainty. This time I clenched my teeth and he seemed less certain. He was smiling less. I watched him chew on the end of a biro, weighing up whether to buy me a fantastic new train set or book tokens. Instead he sent me along the corridor to a woman who inserted much more serious and painful needles. I asked her about the brain tumour, but she wasn't particularly interested. I liked her as well, but at no point did she give me the impression that she was my relative.

It was about an hour later when we walked back in to see Doctor Tiago. He was now seated at a desk fiddling with a piece of paper and this was when Gill noticed that his leg was twitching. Not that he wasn't smiling any more. It's just that on this occasion his frown needed to be displaced elsewhere within his body. In this case, to his right femur and the quadriceps that were supporting it. And this time he had a medical student with him who stood squarely and uprightly by his side, reflecting an air of high rank on Doctor Tiago to which, to his great credit, he seemed entirely unsuited. Because here was his smile again. I wonder if this is all a doctor needs. Just an engulfing smile. Its irradiating and detoxifying effects. He had clearly decided on the train set. Of course! Doctor Tiago would never fob me off with tokens. We were all back together again. But, actually, there wasn't much of an interval between this smile and Doctor Tiago telling me that I had motor neurone disease. Or not that exactly. Not that I had this disease. Just that it would be impossible for it to be anything else. I like that. It's perfect manners when handling bad news. It's not that it's the thing. It's just *not* all the other things.

I had placed motor neurone disease on the same shelf in my brain where I keep the phone number for Dignitas in Switzerland. This was on a high-up shelf in the outhouse with a broken tricycle and an unused bread maker. Immediately prior to receiving the diagnosis I had been slouching in the corridor. I was holding my phone and browsing inanely through online drivel with my thumb. This was just a few moments before.

When I started crying my head was parallel with the desktop. The sob I experienced was just like the deep vibration of a kitchen tap after the mains water is turned back on. A series of metallic shudders through my spine. A chug. A gurgle. And then water. I remember looking up at Gill. She was crying more gently as she looked down at me. I was over her knee by this point, with my neck arched up towards her. And on her face was the shock of sorrow. Not for herself. For me. I will never read a face like that in a moment like that again. It's a wonder to know, that with all the muscular variation the human face is capable of, some permutations are as unique as fingerprints.

We said our goodbyes. Doctor Tiago came out from behind his completely inappropriate desk. His hug confirmed that he was indeed my uncle. I hadn't been imagining this at all. I'm glad that I was diagnosed in Portugal. To be amongst these warm-hearted people. In most other places, doctors seem to belong, or aspire to belong, to the notion of a particular caste or stratum. But doctors in Portugal carry themselves like people who just walked in off the street and put on a white coat. Which is what they are. Which is exactly what all doctors are. It's just that doctors in Portugal appear to know this.

In the corridor, Gill and I ran into Paula, the medical secretary of the neurology department. She'd been expecting us. She stood there in her white coat, with her eyes moist, and her hands clasped as if she was cradling a young chick. I owe a lot to Paula. If it wasn't for Paula, I'd still be limping around the ground floor of Coimbra hospital, somewhere near the impenetrable network of lifts. The Portuguese health system was a little tricky for me to understand. But I had Paula, so I didn't really have to understand anything. By that time in Portugal, after my wife and boys, I'd talk to Paula more than anyone else. She'd push me around the hospital in a wheelchair and drop me at the train station after appointments. For some weeks Paula had been perfecting her version of Leonard Cohen's 'Hallelujah' on the ukulele. She'd been sending me various versions as MP4 files. And now I understood. She'd known about my disease long before Doctor Tiago. I later spoke to her about this and she confirmed my theory to be partially true, but not entirely. In fact, she said that Doctor Tiago knew; he just didn't want to *admit* he knew. It made him feel too sad. Maybe he was better at not knowing than I'd given him credit for. After hearing this, he went up even further in my estimation. I already loved him; there wasn't much further up for him to go.

'You will suffer. You know this, right?'

We'd rented a very old car whilst in Portugal and it had a cassette player. We just regarded it as an artefact and told Tom all about this strange device. And then a month into having the car, Tom was fiddling with the buttons and out popped a cassette. Of fado music. It had been raining all winter and we'd been driving around in the rain playing it ever since – unaware that our car had been thoughtfully preparing us for tragedy. So it felt like we understood this moment. This moment with Paula.

'It will be hard, you know? It will be very hard.'

Paula dropped the tiny chick on the grey-tiled floor.

'You must be happy, Gill. Oh, Gill, you must be strong!'

She cupped Gill's face in her hands.

'Because Joe will be handicapped. His body will stop working. Almost completely. You will see.'

She was a little closer now. Almost nose to nose.

'He will die. You know this, right?'

She took both of us by the hand.

'You must love life. You must be happy!'

As Gill and I staggered along the concourse I felt I had to try and mention this thing about Dignitas. Or something like that. I'm not so brand-orientated that I would have insisted on Dignitas. I needed to admit to this general idea – to spit it out – but it felt like the mains had been turned off again or someone's boot was stuck in the pipe. I was trying to talk. I was trying to cry. My hands were on my knees. I was trying to communicate but only spit came out. A thick, gloopy spit. Down my shirt and all over my trousers. And I was sweating. I was trying to say what I had now just remembered. My Dignitas plan. But Gill was pulling my arm, as if she thought this was not a plan but instead something to do with the piece of tarmac I was standing on. So that if she could pull me away from that spot I would be OK. How unlike tourists we must have seemed in that moment. Pulling and wrenching as doctors and porters and patients in hospital gowns parted around us.

*

Really bad news is a little like medieval weaponry. It isn't precise like a bullet or a machine-sharpened blade. Part of its brute effect comes from blunt power, so that extensive collateral damage is caused to areas already weakened for a variety of other reasons: areas that are sometimes quite a long way beyond the originally intended location. In this sense, they both destroy and clear away. They bring forward endings in a more timely manner – tidying away what had already grown weak. And I think it's not possible to be properly aware of such quiet, broad-reaching devastation, so that it's only discovered later when performing an innocuous task – like reaching for some tinned tomatoes in a cupboard – and you notice some white part of the bone revealed in a place you would have never expected it.

I couldn't have known it at the time, but a lot more became visible to me in the days following my bad news, and I don't think I'm alone in being someone who walks around with all kinds of weaknesses that go back many years – almost as far back as it's possible to go in a life. In the hours after Doctor Tiago diagnosed me I would not have been aware of this, of the soreness and the calcification that had existed for all this time. And that's why the very worst kind of bad news – whilst seeming, of course, really bad – can also perform the same function as a brace applied to wonky teeth, or metal pins through the spine. It can take some time for its brutal benefits to become clear.

When I now look back at that early devastating comprehension of my condition, I see that it was necessary, in a way, to dig and scoop away at an area that should have long ago been knocked through – like a section of blown plaster after a leak; as if this wasn't simply bad news, or advanced notice of a premature end, but also a long-overdue resolution.

*

I spent five days crying. There were intermissions when I could build fantastical, ornate wooden tower blocks with Tom. These periods enabled fresh fluids to be taken in, so that I could begin again at night-time or during the school day. During those nights I awoke several times to cry. Often I had just been dreaming of the diagnosis. And then, sitting up in bed, the expectation was that the day would flow in to dissipate and dissolve. When it didn't, it was as if dreams had lost their function. It was an unschooling of the ways in which bad dreams are meant to be dispersed. Sleep was diminished. And waking was never quite achieved.

I had no previous facility for crying. No track record. I think I could take the image of Doctor Tiago in his white coat and replace it with one in which he wears a white hard-hat. Tiago the Engineer, overseeing a vast hydroelectric power plant. He had pressed a button or pulled a lever, because it began in that moment. It swelled up somewhere from a series of large, loosely fitted metal parts. So that I was just a vessel. A pipe. A tap. A drain. I was not the beginning and not the end. Something is running through me. I'm in the car or lying in bed and all the metal parts of Tiago the Engineer's vast hydroelectric power plant burst and split, and then the water comes.

I now realize what Doctor Tiago and the other neurologists were doing. It was quite an artifice. I admire it now because it helped me a great deal. They dispersed my fears with their wonderful array of smiles. They needed me slouched against walls, bored, complacent. Because if I had been led incrementally towards diagnosis, I would never have gained entry to this vast hydroelectric power plant about which I had never previously been aware. They have to lead you towards it while simultaneously keeping it outside your field of vision. And suddenly, there you are, with other people who've made the same journey. Other recipients of this sudden violence. Perhaps they feel it in other ways: as a conscious fall from a high place or perhaps a sense of having misplaced something important, like the whole universe. In this place of vast latent power and unfathomable depth. And without this place, or outside this place, loss is never really felt. Outside, loss is dispersed, and becomes a kind of unseen haze. But here, down here, it's felt. I found this out. Down here there is nothing but feeling it. The power of it.

I can walk for miles in this underground cavern and remain as I am. And I do. But up above my children are growing older. They're living a life with Gill in a place I don't know. And all the time I can see them from here. A life that works. The boys older. Life happening. I'm not getting closer to any of this. It just gets smaller and darker and fainter as it disappears into the distance. And then the water comes. And then it comes. And it does.

*

I was eating scrambled eggs, watching the milk pump out from Tom's mouth as he spooned up his cereal. It was a natural and effective overflow that meant he didn't have to regulate the amount of milk or cereal he was shovelling in. Gill had her back to us, making packed lunches, and over Tom's shoulder I could see Jimmy trying to mount a sofa that was several hands too high for him. I got up and went through to the bedroom to lie down on my side. I pulled the pillow into my bottom lip and squeezed my face together, wringing it out, so that the pillow became damp around my eye socket. I could hear Gill telling Tom to get his shoes on. Then my diaphragm started chugging. It felt like hiccups but was more rapid and rhythmical. More like a pulsing. I rolled over on to my back and pulled the pillow into my teeth. There's an ambient, wheezing noise that accompanies this kind of sobbing – a layer of treble that makes it sound as though I'm pleading for some kind of mercy. I had a toy once that made this noise when you turned it upside down. It was supposed to sound like a cow, but it was more like a smoker's wheeze. I was tucking my knees into my chest and breathing more steadily now. I heard a door open in the next room, and Gill was stating something assertively. I knew that she was gathering up Tom's schoolbag and I wanted to say goodbye. I could tell the episode was almost over and I sat up on the edge of the bed. This was the functionality of tears that I became used to in those five days. I knew I needed a moment after the exertion, like knowing when I need a cup of tea. I had my hands on my knees and looked around. Nothing had changed. Then I went back into the kitchen.

When the crying came at night, I'd be squeezing the duvet in my fists and thinking very acutely of the physicality of Tom and Jimmy. It must have been something close to focused meditation because I would imagine their current form, then focus in on the changes that I imagined would take place in their bodies in the years to come. I would imagine the lengthening of Tom's lean legs and the broadening of his V-shaped jawline. I imagined the fine, fair hair that would appear on his face. I imagined his length and strength and the cheekbones that would one day underline his gaze. With Jimmy, I love and marvel at the width of his feet and hands. I imagine him continuing to be broad and solid. His shoulders would thicken and his jawline would be rounder than Tom's. I imagined him shorter than Tom but more burly. In Jimmy's case I also felt guilt that I knew his physical shape and form, but that he would never remember mine. He would often nap on the bed with his chin cupped in his hands and I would talk to his sleeping body and tell him how sorry I was.

Over the Portuguese winter it rained continuously in the mountains, and the eucalyptus that burnt all summer now smelt green. Descending the mountain, we'd wind down through these forests and the warm microclimate inside the car created ideal conditions for precipitation. Any thought or awareness or reflection simply switched it on. The road snaked and seemed to further dislodge all the salty snotty liquid within. I could have leant forward and found the button on the dashboard. And it would come, rising up through the pipes pooling inside my head. Then I'd hit the button again and it would stop.

During those days it felt like some figure was cutting around me with a pair of scissors; moving me with the blades to cut close and accurately. And as the paper turned, more of me would drop down and I knew that it wouldn't take long for the scissors to have made their whole way round. I would be imagining the boys and Gill. Living in a place I might not know – a life that worked but which was alien to me. The boys older. Life happening. And I was looking at all of this from the outside. I clung to Gill, but I saw her and Tom and Jimmy connected by something that I wasn't. They seemed somehow in place and as they should be. And though I was holding on, I wasn't connected in the same way. Until this time I'd just assumed that we were formed from a single piece. That something like this could never happen. A little family of four pinched into human form and then hardened. Set. Finished. So that one figure could never be the person outside observing all these parts. That it would necessarily become a complete form made up of three figures is one of the things I dis-covered in this cavernous place. This is a concept that I looked at and looked at and looked at and looked at again and again, and I could not understand it. And all the moments that had upset me in the past were in one place. And this moment of upset was in another place. It was an entire physical feeling. And when it came my body curled inwards like a fortune-telling fish on a hot palm.

*

When the five days of tears came they filled the spaces I had never known. Unused rooms. Forgotten rooms. The places where I might have been. It crashed through barriers and washed away impediments like they were blades of grass. It carried me away – it carried everything away. I bobbed on the surface of this rising, moving water, my arms outstretched – a little man being carried away. There was no need to call out; there was no other way to travel; only water. Nothing was left behind. No selves in tiny corners, no scary thoughts left buried. A bowl of chocolate ice cream, which I ate when I was five, went by upon the surface of the flood. A teacher half remembered, a scrap of brown carpet, the car I crashed when I was seventeen, a painted wooden block – all bobbing in the water along with me.

At the end of those five days the water seeped back into the ground and the emotions left behind were those that I had never allowed myself to fully know or really feel: vulnerability for what I was and am and will become. Very simple feelings. I've had conversations about the value of laughter, but I no longer believe it is the best medicine. At the end of my five days of crying, I felt calmer and more at ease than at any time in my life. I could have held out my hand and weighed myself in my palm and guessed exactly to a gram the scale of this little life of mine. I knew myself in those dark days. I felt quieter. I listened to the loss and knew exactly where and who I was. It felt like a gift. Extremely small, yet conspicuous against a dark background. Like something reclaimed.

Cuckmere Haven

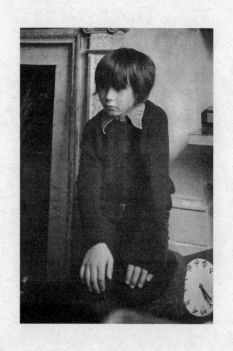

When we arrived, the land around this white-clad Welsh farmhouse seemed flat and overrun. Long grass sprouted in the vegetable patches next to a rusting red tractor, tilting into the ground. And strewn across this wide, unkempt area were the remains of various long-disused bicycles.

This was the late 1970s and I was eight or nine years old. The house was something to do with my mum's boyfriend at the time and he was taking her there for the weekend. I was travelling down with them in the rear of his VW camper, staring out at the M4 between the backs of their heads.

The interior of this communal household was shabby, with fabric throws and decrepit painted wooden furniture. The house smelt fetid with incense and things left unwashed – like something coming to an end. Several families lived there and a few, like us, were just passing through, but I didn't form a connection with the other children. For the days of our stay I largely played in the garden with a bicycle rim or sat in the camper reading comics. But on both mornings I was up early and came down to the warm kitchen where a huge side of communal bacon hung from a piece of cord. It looked very different from the bacon we kept in a packet in our fridge and I'd watch people taking to it with a knife. It was shredded and ragged and I remember I found it so grotesque I couldn't stop looking at it. Various wonky-looking people would come down for breakfast and slice what they wanted. I didn't know what we were doing in this house, and no one said very much, so I stationed myself on a stool in one corner of the kitchen watching the hanging piece of meat sway to a standstill.

The other clear memory I have is of going to sleep with five or six other children in a large double bed. I don't think this was in any way a playful experience or something fun, because I remember the moments before bedtime and the panicked visual search for better options – like the search for a tree root when sliding off a cliff. I was feeling uncomfortably wedged in and wishing that I was one of the children on the edge of the bed. I was surprised by the situation, but I can't recall if I saw the night through or if I found an alternative for the second night. Though at least eight years old, I was still wetting my bed, so I imagine this was a large part of my reluctance.

On one of the days, all the adults took magic mushrooms together and everyone got into various vehicles and set off to the beach. It was a pebble beach at high tide, in autumn or winter. It's possible I might have noticed changes in people's behaviour but I'm not sure. We were just a collection of people going to the beach for the afternoon. I have no recollection of my feelings at the time – quite the opposite, in fact – only what happened in the moments after we arrived. I didn't join the others; I didn't walk down on to the beach – I just stood there looking down at the group on the beach. I only remember the adults, but there may have been children – there must have been because it was a large group of people; I just know I wasn't with them. I was standing apart from the others on a bank about twenty feet above, on a shallow cliff of sand and stone.

I had gathered stones in my hand and I was looking down at them. They were a mixture of blues and creamy shades of speckled eggshell. A few moments later I started throwing my carefully selected stones at the group and I noticed that the blue flat ones seemed to arc and zip through the air, so that they landed with some speed and unpredictability. I could loop them upwards or sideways but, whichever way I threw them, the men and women below would sway or jump, flicking their heels behind them like nervy colts. I wasn't conscious of wanting to hit anyone and I didn't go chasing anyone with the stones. It was more mesmeric than this.

In the first few moments there was a lot of confusion and, from what I now know, I think what they had collectively taken would have made it hard for these people to establish what was real or imagined. But as they became more aware of my presence, and kept their eyes fixed on the trajectory of the stones, they were able to part like schools of fish. And they would alternate between evasive measures and the heightening ferocity of the way they addressed me; the snarling of their features and the shouts they made – the tearing shapes they made with their mouths. And then it stopped or I imagine it stopped. I don't know how this ended. I have no recollection; just of the throwing and the people below. And that was it.

*

Even though the world appears to be still, when looking up at birds circling overhead it can feel even more still in comparison to what's above. So that if you crane your neck upwards for any length of time, at some pigeons or a pair of kites or, as in this case, seagulls – your tongue feels heavy in your throat and something giddying happens, as if the rotating planet has inadvertently revealed itself. You might even tip back at the base of the neck, or feel that you are about to, until you stretch your arms out sideways and take a balancing step backwards, your tongue loosening and your throat softening, as you steady yourself on the even more stationary world.

When the piece of carpet and the bowl of chocolate ice cream floated by, so did this boy, but largely forgotten and still up on that cliff with stones in hand, after all this time. And now it feels like such a simple thing to go up there and take his much smaller hand in mine or just to stand up there with him for a time, looking out at what he can see. We might even forget about those people below, as if they never existed. I don't know what we'd do – just something that felt comfortable for this little boy. It seems so simple to me; such a simple action. To come down from this place after such a long time.

We'd come home; I'd tell my sons to budge up on the sofa. We'd wrap him up in blankets and then carry on as normal – just doing things and reading books and cooking and playing and arguing over whether it's one or two biscuits. The same things that we always do but with this other person present, as if he always had been.

*

Three years before the stones upon the cliff, my parents had been in the process of separating. From what I remember, people in that house lived quite separately and there was often a lot of shouting at night, so that by the time we did come to leave I don't think I was disappointed.

I suppose this home had shared a particular feature with the homes of all unhappy families. If you enter any of these places and climb the stairs, you'll find on the top step at least one breakfast-bowl-size indentation in the carpet: one central indentation for homes with an only child, one more for each child between the ages of four and twelve. It's where the children perch in their nightwear, elbows propped on knees, hands holding up saggy faces, silently absorbing the shrieky, spitty ping-pong of Mummy and Daddy's complaints below.

I can record most of what I heard from the top step because the same script played out again and again for both of them, at intervals of between one and three years, with so many different partners. So they just went on from this situation, spinning and spinning into other relationships that ended with the same unhappiness.

My mum was in her mid thirties, tall and pretty, with long straight dark hair. Her face and neck gave the impression of being somewhat elongated, or stretched, and angled ever so slightly upwards, as if this aspect of her body was trying unsuccessfully to get away from something objectionable lying on the ground. She was a little skittish and nervous but, in her relationships with men, there always seemed to be a random moment when one too many outrages would send her spiralling and shrieking, like one of those circular fireworks that spray out sparks from a standing position, in all kinds of directions.

I think at this point in their lives they were both having affairs and upsetting each other with some abandon, and there seemed to be some mutually enforceable night-time dance in which the full details of each other's betrayals gave vent to what was most combustible. One of the strange features in my father's character was that these were the only occasions in which he would properly grin and let other people see his teeth. He was swarthy with deep-set blue eyes, and long dark hair that he'd often stroke backwards from his brow, and with his pursed mouth he had developed a brooding, noirish demeanour. It was fairly subtle at this stage in his life – and he was just a few years older than my mum – but as he aged, and had more dental work done, or when his gums naturally receded, he had to make a conscious effort, when smiling, to pull his top lip down as far as possible over his dentures.

If they'd known, or orchestrated their rows more effectively, they could have written their rants down on cards and held them up to their squablees, and that way they wouldn't have needed to wake me up. Because these complaints were always the same, the pleading was always the same – to anyone, to everyone. The spitting and shrieking at each other, at the skies, for some kind of attention or some kind of distance. And wondering why nobody is listening. These must have been such ancient voices, so that the two small eyes peering down through the balusters were really no smaller or more frightened than the ones below.

So that one could have complained and the other shouted, 'Snap!'

Or that they could have written down their complaints, cut them up, placed them upside down in rows, knelt together on the carpet and played matching pairs.

Or made snow globes out of each complaint and shaken them at each other.

*

I think a terminal diagnosis is the very finest tool a writer can have; it's the view from an escarpment of both the beginning and the end. It's rare to be able to see along the stretch of a landscape, so that nothing exists in isolation, but is seen instead as part of a wide sweeping single entity of land. And objects, or moments, which have long floated in vast pools of memory, suddenly become visible and re-formed and completely still.

Before we had children, Gill and I used to walk the Sussex Downs and all along the coastal paths. Even when we moved to London, we'd sometimes get up early on a Sunday and travel down for breakfast by the sea. The place we'd park was Seaford. We'd lace up our boots on the benches, looking out at the waves, and then ascend the first of many high-up undulating chalky cliffs. From the very top we'd glance across and see the Seven Sisters, and once or twice we'd walk these higher cliffs, but this was our place. This series of climbs and descents between a beachfront car park and a broad pebble expanse where the flood plains of Cuckmere Haven spill out into the sea. We'd walk in rain and sun and pulverize ourselves with wind and sea, along this giant carved out stretch of chalk. And even more than that: the single cliff, part way along the walk, which offers both a glimpse, not only of the end, but also of the start. The place where we had parked and the long, wide beach where we would eat our lunch. Looking ahead and knowing where it finishes; looking behind and seeing where it started.

There is a photo of five-year-old me, standing in the garden in grey shorts and a maroon T-shirt. My crooked knees are covered by my hands. I look ready for something. I look eager. And below this, an arrow drawn in red biro picks out the blond-haired Action Man at my feet.

Apart from time spent at the top of the stairs, I have two further memories from this period. The first is the discovery that I could make my own ice cream by melting two different flavours and returning them to the freezer. The second is coming into the living room and seeing every piece of furniture turned upside down. The floor strewn with spillages and books and vases and anything that had once stood upright now crooked or broken or on the floor. Not a single item in the room remained as it should be.

*

After my parents separated, I would visit my father every other weekend. The family home had been given up and he'd rented a small bungalow on a main residential street not far from where we once had lived. Sometimes I'd sit on the front wall and watch a group of older shirtless boys who'd cycle up and down, no-handed, with perfectly upright postures. There was a large garden with a pond and a large living room where I would spend my Saturday visits eating sweets and watching TV. There were several women who came and went, but the one I remember was tall and bony, with a tight blonde perm.

Arriving one weekend, I noticed a hole in the unpainted living-room door, a fresh, deep dent about a quarter way up: the kind of hole you might make if you were to take a normal-sized hammer and swing it upwards very hard. I think my father laughed about it and what he told me in this moment was that the woman had tried to kick him. I believed this – not only because I was five, and believed what people told me, but also because I found her terrifying.

On one of these Saturdays I was lying on the living-room sofa watching the wrestling on *World of Sport* when this tall woman landed over the threshold of the room. Her movements were stilted and angular, as if she were hopping rather than walking. Her neck jerked uncomfortably left and right, and she appeared to be looking for something quite specific, but then she changed angles and diverted towards me. I suppose she must have been carrying a lot of tension, and that something must have happened, because once she arrived at the sofa she picked up one of the cushions and threw it at my head. I imagine, for a moment, that the two of us might have watched the cushion bounce away and watched it come to a stop on the carpeted floor, but if there was any peace, or a release for her in this moment, it seemed to pass quickly because she then bent her knees and, as she screeched, thrust out a kind of jazz-hands movement –

as if this was her nest, as if her wingspan was vast, as if she'd landed here from another epoch and found that I'd eaten all her eggs – which I can understand would have been quite distressing. But at the time I didn't know what this was. I took my feet down from the sofa, in case that's what it was. It wasn't clear at all. She just made this sound, without even looking at me, and then she left. It was the not knowing that confused me. It was a little bit more frightening because of that. So when I visited I was very careful about what I said or did.

She was the first I can remember of the women in his life from this time. Over about a ten-year period he must have found all of his girlfriends at the top of a very steep precipice and then continued going to this very same location to retrieve new ones. I imagine they may have been quite willing, given how frightening it must have been up there. I spent time with so many of them, from the age of five until I was fifteen, and they always seemed to be on the edge of something – of violence or despair or alcoholism, or all of these and perhaps some other things too. There was a common feeling of vulnerability and volatility, and I wonder what it was that he felt he needed from the sadness of these lives.

*

One of the great challenges facing children is that they're always having to glance upwards at adults and, at a very young age, this angle can be considerable. It's always so much better to be able to assess objects or people from a more or less level position. It's a particular problem for children when the adults around them are tilting and swerving in a trajectory that carries significant amounts of risk. From their lower position to the ground it's just not possible for children to properly assess the level of risk that higher-up individuals are subjecting themselves to and, by virtue of their proximity, the children in their care. This is why children are so vulnerable to those who exploit angular advantage for malign intent, or who do so because they are not, and never have been, and never will be, in safe control of their own altitude.

In the final few weeks in Portugal, Tom and Jimmy's view of adult life had been delightfully skewed by our precipitous placement on the side of a mountain. When the bread van parked outside at 2 p.m. they reached up to the baker through his rolled-down window to each receive a fresh bread roll. And when our car wouldn't start Gill managed to mime this action to four old men playing cards in the street. A few minutes later a tiny red tractor arrived with jump leads, and its arrival was treated with such awe by Tom and Jimmy. This key-turning mime had made Gill a local celebrity, and it seemed that it wasn't just the gesture but the pathetic churning gurning sound that accompanied it. Across the village we were then universally greeted with a beaming smile, and the signature facsimile of Gill's famous *air ignition*. A few nights into this newfound attention, we opened the front door and four village women stood on our doorstep asking Gill to come dancing with them. They giggled a little, looking sideways at each other, before spilling into each other's shoulders in a bobbing motion and, whilst gyrating their hips and knees, demonstrated – through the repeated joyous rotation of their thumbs and forefingers – that Gill's ignition mime had now become an established dance move.

*

My father's house burnt down and he rented a flat with long corridors that had once been a retirement home. It had the fragrance of grandparents and chrome room numbers still attached to the doors. I believe I was still five, perhaps six, and he had a tall, dark-haired girlfriend, who was just nineteen years old. I don't know, but I wonder if he felt prompted to be more active during this period, because of her youthfulness. In the evenings they were often at the pub, playing darts. Depending on the pub, sometimes I'd get a knock on the car window, which was always very exciting, and I'd be allowed to sit just behind the door with a packet of crisps. It was a period of time when he was also covered in rich, purple bruises all over his neck, chest, arms and back. I imagined they were painful and I was worried by them.

In that flat I remember a bedroom at the very end of the long, main corridor. I was particularly interested because it was inside this room that I first discovered a stack of porn, stored in a painted green rattan box at the end of the bed. In the mid 1970s, porn magazines were a slightly more conspicuous part of life, or so it seemed to me. They had yet to be completely consigned to the top shelf in newsagent's and I remember it seemed to be quite normal.

Even though I was shocked when I finally got to see inside one of these magazines, and even though I struggled with the images, something always made me go back. There were a few occasions over the years when my father caught me with them and he always seemed to feel aggrieved or wronged – as if something had been done to him.

It was more common for this pique to ignite in response to something that one of his girlfriends had done or not done, like something not being cooked the way he'd wanted. I remember his clipped eruption and the way his arms would move wildly as he exited the room. I would freeze, looking straight ahead, so that with my peripheral vision I'd witness the thrashing swim-stroke movement of his arms – his angry slapping backstroke – across the living room and out into the hallway, shouting about the ingredients as he went, and the sense that he would have departed more rapidly, and with greater dignity, were he not having to wrench each foot out and lift each knee to free himself from some claggy kind of mud. It would have been silent for some time after that. This was the pattern. No one would have spoken and then he would have returned some minutes or hours later.

There was one Sunday on which a table had been set outside. I think the actual living-room table had been brought out into the garden and the dishes clinked and clonked as we all served ourselves. There was a lot of focus and not much conversation. And then my father asked about the gravy.

Reflecting on this incident now, I think the most likely reason for the absence of gravy was perhaps the inexperience of the cook. I can't quite remember which of the girlfriends he was with at the time. I can't quite picture her, but I remember she'd gone to a lot of effort because it all looked quite good to me. I imagine her mistake in this situation was entirely benign and that she had thought of almost everything.

He sank back in his chair: this gravy business seemed to be a really terrible oversight for him. Really disappointing. I think the sight of the dry ingredients was a little too much for him and he pushed his plate away. You could tell there was a sense of injustice about this situation; the last straw or something, and I think he said as much. And I was feeling bad for him because I always did. The twisting of his familiar features, the contorted, distorted anger of it all. And I would look away, or down, waiting for it all to finish, waiting for an object to be broken, waiting for what he had to say, about gravy or something. Waiting for him to walk away and for the next day when everyone could start speaking again.

Some time after the girl who was nineteen, there was an older woman in his life. She had a daughter of about my age called Kelly, and I froze when I first saw someone my own size in this house. I think we both did, but then she turned and flapped like a goose in take-off and trotted down the corridor, as if the bottom half was pony. And right until the moment when it ended so suddenly, about three months later, I don't think there was ever any point when I wouldn't have followed her at speed along the corridor.

I remember once discovering a collection of canes and whips. I asked around for why they were there, but no one would give me an answer. Then someone asked me why I thought we had so many older male visitors. I couldn't answer that: I just added this to my void, which I now know to be the useful repository for all unhappy children. And I don't exactly remember Kelly's mum and whether this collection of objects had been hers, or whether she had been one of the other women he knew over these years who did this kind of work, but whatever the situation I think that was a confusing household for a child and I don't think the available clues made it straightforward for Kelly or me to work it out.

*

We're now several months into Tom's subscription to *Land Rover Monthly*. The third copy arrived two days ago and Gill and I are taking it in turn to read with Tom about reconditioned crankshafts and timing-belt adjustment kits. Last night we learnt all about the second-generation P38 Range Rover and, in particular, that landmark moment in 1994 when the transition from the old 200Tdi to the new 300Tdi brought with it an added level of refinement to the torque and acceleration of the P38.

I've noticed that Gill is as prone as I am to sliding *Land Rover Monthly* behind the backs of sofa cushions, or slightly higher on the bookshelves than Tom might be able to reach. But just before seven, whatever we have done, a copy emerges and we begin this night-time read without any of us understanding anything technically more specific than *engine* or *wheel*.

However hard I find these passages are to read, I look at Tom's face – its implacable adherence to these inscrutable texts – and I realize my discomfort is of such insignificance compared to the consuming effort of Tom's endeavour. Something tiny is located deep within these monthly magazines that lies buried several miles underground, and we are all searching for it, despite none of us knowing what it is. Or if it *does* exist. But that doesn't matter – its veracity or otherwise. Tom shines his powerful torch at the soil and Gill and I lend our hands to turn over the earth, using our fingers to sift for secrets that may or may not be present.

I recognize the burrowing of my six-year-old son. Every parent recognizes this work that children undertake. And even as he sits on my lap, my eyes are also watching from a quiet dark corner on the other side of the room, and peacefully observing this lonely universal search of a child, and understanding, and feeling that it's all OK, and that perhaps it always was.

*

When I think of any children's play, whether that's playing Mums and Dads or anything else, I think of the pure oblivion that takes place, so that you could be an adult walking through the field of play and not a single child would register your presence in that moment. Whether that play takes place away from the adult gaze, or out in the open, it won't affect the quality of what's taking place, or that necessary feeling of immersion for those children involved. And when Kelly suggested she was Mum and I was Dad, the bedroom must have offered some of the architectural experience of domesticity, to which we probably added crockery and cutlery and other props. But I think the door was always closed, and we didn't quite experience that oblivion in the moment, so that we might have checked the whereabouts of adults when we played – we might have wandered up the corridor, or into the garden, just to check. And then we'd come back, and it didn't take long in the history of our play to think of the bed as being something vital in what we were trying to work out, and to think that our clothes may have been far less vital, or perhaps some kind of impediment.

I imagine this sense of oblivion is really important when trying things out through play, and maybe that's an essential part of what makes it enjoyable. As our play developed in this propless way, I know that we smiled less and that some of the chatter we had grown to expect became much reduced once we had taken all our clothes off. It's not just children, but adults too, who stop talking when actions become unsafe. And I didn't see much need to speak because Kelly had a much clearer idea of how this game was played. Because I was six I didn't question why a girl of five would be quite so determined to achieve this end, in a game like this, or how she would have gleaned the rules for the way the pieces of the game were set up. I would take my own clothes off, but I couldn't bring myself to watch or be active in what we were doing. I tended to be draping my arms back over my head as if I was looking for something behind me or perhaps that my hat had fallen off and I was using all my fingers to reach for it – looking up and searching for as long as I needed to or until the whole thing came to an end.

And that was it – from playing Mums and Dads, to this. I think about this time and wonder if the games of other boys and girls would ever lead to this. I'm sure it's possible, but I think, more often, the minds of five- and six-year-olds don't get to this. But I don't know; just that ours did.

After we were caught for the terrible and selfish thing we did, I don't remember us playing very much together, and it wasn't long before Kelly and her mum moved on. I missed my gap-toothed friend as much as I have ever missed anyone in my life. And I have always

— 83 —

remembered her and spent my life worrying about her – hoping that she is now OK and, perhaps, that she forgives me for the awful wrong I must have committed, whatever that may have been.

*

We're all sleeping in one bedroom, in a cottage on a farm in rural Hampshire. It's all bed in here and very little floor – so that we might as well be in the desert somewhere in a tent, under the stars. But it's rainy and windy and both Tom and Jimmy are asleep in their beds: their bodies stretching out – their peaceful, working, breathing, sleeping bodies. I like to come in here and feel my restless breathing sinking into theirs. This room at night-time – the wind rattling the iron roof on the barn, the mice scratching behind the skirting boards. The rain falling from the guttering and the snort of a two-year-old as he runs his arm towards his head, turning his hand outwards and upwards like the movement of a small turbine, tilting him over and on to his back.

Everywhere is now a vantage point – looking back at the past from a clifftop and the trajectory of flat stones fizzing towards a group of hippies on a beach or, here, looking down at my sleeping children and being close enough to feel the heat from the rising and falling of their bodies. But I don't think I see any more clearly now, it's just that everything has become more visible against the background. What's behind is now filled in with a pale watery wash so that it's easier to pick out detail in everything, from the foreground right up to the horizon. It's always been there but I see it now; it's not floating around in space any more. It's returning to the body, descending out of the free-floating darkness and settling into place.

*

After the separation, and as my father moved into the place where all these women came and went, my mum had found a cottage in a village. The pretty little house was near the end of an unmade road, backing on to an open meadow with a stream. It had a garden with an apple orchard, a damson tree and a stone bust of a regal-looking woman, accented with lichen, with half an ear and no nose. She stood in a flower bed by the front gate, circled by a narrow, paved walkway – sometimes with a cat upon her head and sometimes in the rain.

At first, I liked this house and lived a certain kind of life, in which I was a little man. I felt much more relaxed here and not scared in the way I was at my father's. There were two places set for dinner and, next to the front passenger seat in the car, a little tray where

I could keep all my belongings: my pen, two cars, toy soldiers, a piece of useful plastic and several conkers. At night I'd listen to stories about a monkey called Alfonso and in the morning I'd run into my mum's bedroom and play disappearing mountains on her knees. And before long a lazy weekend would have passed, or we'd travel to friends, or I'd accompany her to parties. I fell in love in a conscious way – for the very first time.

On the first occasion when a boyfriend came and stayed, he laid the table differently. We went for a drive together in the car and I scooped the contents from my tray in the front and kept them on my lap in the back. A week or two would pass and maybe he would stay again. I let him lay the table and found a plastic bucket for my belongings in the car. In the morning I decided not to run in and jump on my mum; instead I looked through a book and waited for their footsteps. After that, he came a few more times and then it stopped.

One day I asked about this man. I was sitting next to my mum at the dinner table – just the two of us – and I was told he wouldn't be staying again. I was pleased with this news and agreed with her that it wouldn't be a good idea to have him back in our house. I agreed with her list of complaints. We both were of the same mind and I was delighted to hear my mum say that, in any case, she always found me better company. Everything seemed clear and I returned the contents of my plastic bucket to the tray in the front passenger side of the car.

Several months later a different man came to stay. I was a little disappointed to find that we were in the same situation again, but I set the table the way the man before had laid it and went to check the location of my plastic bucket. It had only been a few months and I remembered how the evening used to go. This time, I paid close attention to what this man had to say and tried to make a judgement about which of us had been the better company that evening. He didn't seem anything special and I was fairly sure he wouldn't be back again. Unfortunately, a few days later, he came to stay again. And a few times over the next month the same thing happened. On one occasion things were said at the table that reminded me a little of some of the things I used to hear when I would sit at the top of the stairs in our old house. I particularly noticed the way my mum, after the meal was finished, made a lot of noise with the cutlery as she put it, quite vigorously, into the washing-up bowl.

It was a surprise to me that this same man continued coming to the house. My mum didn't seem very happy and I was allowed to eat dinner on my lap, watching television. When he wasn't here I would say a lot of things about the situation that seemed to make sense to her. And then we'd have a treat to cheer us both up or we'd stay up late and watch a film together.

I think I felt a bit annoyed when this man came to stay again. And when the two of them started laughing at the dinner table, about something I didn't understand, I scooped up my plate, my knife and fork and went outside, setting my place down on the shallow paving alongside the regal-looking stone bust in the garden. I gazed up at her and she looked the same as she did that first day when I walked through the garden gate. I thought about this and, eating my way through the length of my fish finger, considered her constancy and her unblinking eyes. A year or two went by and I think, by this time, I'd lost any pleasure or trust in what I had felt. I'd think more about this woman made of stone and what she had to say to me – and how she somehow mattered more than anyone I knew.

A different man would come to stay – or then he wouldn't. From this point on, I'd always ask to eat my meal upon my lap. I wasn't sure about the quality of my conversation and played with various thoughts – like who exactly my mother did like best – until the blood ran from my eyes and everywhere. I decided to keep my belongings permanently in the plastic bucket and let other people set the knives and forks for dinner – losing my interest in what would happen. I divided my time between this house and weekends at my father's – researching what exactly relationships were from the clues his magazines half gave me. Some time spent there; some time spent here.

And, by the age of nine, found myself on top of a shallow cliff by the sea, throwing stones at the people below.

Losses

The incremental changes to my body is a story that sits on my windowsill in spring and requires repotting every few weeks. It's exciting for the writer and the gardener in me but terrifying for the person that I am. My body is not the same as it was on that cold January day at Three Bridges station. I now spend my time in a wheelchair and keep a note of the tiny little losses; the places I could reach last week that are now out of reach. The simple activities that now challenge me. So much is new and surprising. Last week, a box of tissues stood just out of reach, and I found myself blowing my nose on the non-buttered side of a slice of granary bread, left over from a cheese sandwich.

Not all losses are equal. For example, I now notice that my willy is shrinking. Its absence reminds me of those breeds of dogs who possess just far too much skin for the surface of their body; dogs that somehow seem smaller for all the excess rolls of skin jostling for space on their undersized frames. Or I look down and my shrinking willy reminds me of a once-impressive termite mound, now long abandoned and crumbling from the top.

The reason that I now pee into a bottle is, in part, because it's hard for me to get to the toilet: hard for me to get up, to turn, to manoeuvre, and then to approach. But it's equally the result of the unsettling and unaccountable multi-speed functioning of my urethra. For some reason the waste liquid exiting down my urethra now travels at varying speeds. I can't rely on the family saloon that I had come to know because, without any sighting in my wing mirror, a streaking yellow Lamborghini of piss suddenly passes and sends my flabby concertinaed willy circling wildly like an out-of-control fire hose. As soon as I've finally taken back control, it can seem like the traffic has suddenly stopped; as if the highway has been closed without notice until, a few moments later, a series of elderly cyclists pass me in the slow lane and continue, for what seems like several hours, parting only occasionally to allow through a Kawasaki superbike or a diesel tanker.

*

Between November and February the winter skies were clear and blue. These were the early months following diagnosis and, in the middle of the day, the land around our mountainside cottage was temperate and peaceful. By 11 a.m. on most days I could pull open the sliding doors, limp along to a chair and table by a lemon tree, and set up my laptop under an awning with views over the Rabaçal valley in central Portugal.

It's now November of the following year and Gill, Tom, Jimmy and I are all living in a small rented cottage in the Hampshire countryside. It's 4 p.m., but I don't mind that it's dark and rainy outside. This is a different life. The citrus trees are now oak and ash and yew – and the way I manoeuvre my body to be able to write is a bit like manoeuvring fruit in a lemon squeezer to extract the remaining juice. I can't just sit in a chair and write because I can't *sit* in a chair; more accurately, I can't get out of a chair. My hip flexors no longer flex, my knees give way and both my quadriceps and hamstrings have atrophied. It would take a hoist or two strong people to get me out of a chair.

Before moving to Portugal we lived in a two-bedroom flat in Crystal Palace. With clear skies, and a less-than-average tangerine smog over the London skyline, this southern highpoint offered views across to Alexandra Palace on the northern side of the city. Our flat was on the top floor and from our kitchen and living room we looked out over the city in the distance, with views of

St Paul's and the Shard. For the five miles or so between us and the Thames, mature trees largely obscured the dense housing so that the whole of south London appeared to be forest.

In spring our bungalow will be ready, just thirty minutes east of here, with the vast ash tree at the foot of the garden and the woods beyond. The doors are being widened and hoists are being installed; an extra bed-room's being added and a glass-fronted extension, through which I'll be able to look out at the woods. My aim is to complete this book by then. My left hand functions much as it always has, but there are furrows between the bones of my right hand. When I tap with my index finger, the middle and ring fingers droop and drag along unwanted keys. The trick is to plant the fleshy base of my hands just below the keys and pivot my fingers into place.

It's been the most exciting of adventures – from London to Portugal and back to here. But I don't know if my body will last until this final move. Seven months ago we lived on top of a mountain in a foreign land and now we have come back down again.

*

Given that I can now pee into a bottle, my multi-speed urethra isn't that much of a problem, but other changes feel less easy to adapt to. I'm now uncomfortable at night and find it shocking to approach bedtime with a level of dread.

But once thudded down, and Gill cups my legs to lift them on to the bed, there's very little movement I can make. I'm like a beetle on my back. Less than a mammal. I hear Gill breathing in the night and Jimmy snorting in his cot. I don't feel I am part of this or even part of what's happening in the barn outside or in the field – the resting and the rebuilding, the turning and moving. The way a hoof points downwards in a stretch, one paw curls around another, a hand bends upwards and pushes back the moon. I want to slide my palm along the sheet and bury it under my pillow, or weave the body from the ends of my feet, twisting my legs like two reeds until my torso flips and I'm over on to my front.

These simple, unconsidered actions are now the movements in the mind. Awake at 3 a.m. – imagining the action of sitting up in bed, the soles of the feet touching down on the cold floor. The simplicity of this – sitting with the palms of my hands just resting on my knees. Or moving in the dark – and the luxury of being able to pull the cord on the bathroom light and lift the toilet seat for a pee.

*

I read the words *emerging quadriplegia* in my physio-therapy report and was reminded that I was once an *emerging* playwright and that others are *emerging* foot-ballers. It's aspirational, with status connotations.

With my left hand I still aspire to scratch my own itches. Or I can at least move enough to rub an itch against another limb or the leg of a chair or bed. And if paralysis was once an exotic horror, it's less so now. Being horrified would require me to be unfamiliar, but my body has already given me too much information for this. It's no stretch for me to imagine quadriplegia or to imagine the friendly fly that will one day land on me – feeling each of its six dainty legs on my skin; being patient with the fly, as if the invitation had been mine.

But quadriplegia does feel harsher than paralysis. A person can be paralysed at the waist, either up or down, and lead a perfectly adequate quality of life. Emerging quadriplegia feels like a much more advanced and spe-cialist concept than emerging paralysis; or much more complete. And the more Latinate *quadriplegia* also feels ancient and antique – the egg spilled on my T-shirt, the belly bump and shrunken willy, the toes now curling into claws – that all of this may someday be cast in stone by Michelangelo and placed upon a bed-like plinth within a small museum.

With all the wealth of human civilization making sense of death, quadriplegia is a special kind of loneliness. I need to start being happy in my own skin.

*

When I'm not writing I'd like to say I spend my time reading, listening to opera and learning to meditate; whereas I actually fill my time bingeing on catch-up TV and flicking through social media. Just a few days ago I was surprised to find a very enjoyable film about the experience of having motor neurone disease. It was a violent film: lots of shooting and bloodshed.

The plot involves the exchange of arms between a dealer and a member of the IRA. Each man has his entourage and the ninety minutes of 'real-time' action takes place entirely within a disused warehouse. The film is nothing but guns, a constant flow of witty dialogue and the juxtaposition of a very tender John Denver soundtrack alongside images of wounding and mutilation. About twenty minutes in, a shot is fired, which develops into a firefight that consumes the remainder of the film, grievously maiming all the characters in the story.

The reason this is most certainly a film about motor neurone disease is to do with the type and intensity of wounds inflicted and experienced. No one in this film dies quickly. Many of the wounds inflicted as a result of the environment are just as painful and damaging as gunshot. A person crawls to avoid a bullet and puts his hand and forearm into broken glass. Everything about that wound – its pain and discomfort – is recognized in this moment. And it's these incremental woundings that gradually break down each individual. Towards the end of the film, each character appears chronically, cumulatively and comprehensively disabled. They cannot walk; they cannot crawl. They propel themselves slowly across the gritty floor using shoulders or a chin or whichever minor part of the body feels the least affected by their plight.

There is a resignation in all of these characters. They joke and shout across the space to their dying fellow enemy, knowing that nothing about the present situation can be changed; knowing that they will die and released to accept these final moments with a fuller sense of the character that has falteringly supported them throughout their able-bodied life thus far. They're not different; nor do they tell fewer jokes – they're just weak and dying.

*

I was sat on the side of the bed when a district nurse passed me a mug of tea, which I then dropped into my lap and burnt my testicles.

What strikes me most is that, once this had happened, I was unable to do anything to make the situation better. And I think about my inability to escape a burning building when the time comes. Or if something or someone I love is snatched and I have to watch them getting smaller from my chair as they are taken away from me.

I had been sitting on the side of my bed when I put my hands out and watched my fingers slither and wobble away in the handle of the mug.

And with the shock of that moment my torso fell back as if I were an egg that someone had tried to balance on its end; my feet still on the floor but my eyes on the ceiling and, all the time, my testicles burning because emptying boiling water on to your lap when you're wearing jogging bottoms is like using a flannel as a hot compress.

My wife came running, holding Jimmy in her arms, and a lot of different manoeuvres happened in these moments. I was shrieking at this point, physically unable to do the thing I needed to – which was to pull my trousers away from my testicles. Only in that moment can a person grasp the thermal properties of a pair of jogging bottoms.

By now, Jimmy was also screaming and these nurses (there were two of them, in fact) tried sparking up a conversation with Gill about the best formation and approach (given that my trousers now needed to be pulled down) for preserving my dignity. It's so hard to offer reassurance when shrieking and if they'd known me better they would have been less concerned by this. If they'd known me a year ago, their concerns would have been a lot more relevant.

Once levered to my feet, a towel was placed in front and behind, like a magician holding a square piece of red silk in front of a top hat. Or at the beach – the way a mum might look away as she holds a towel for her teenage son to change behind.

The second time I fell backwards on to the bed (after the manoeuvre was complete) it was laughter that propelled me. As much as I would rather be able to hold my own tea or pull scalding clothes from my body, I'm also hourly reminded that my predicament is chock-full of the indignities that make the experience both entertaining and, more than this, tolerable.

*

I now receive a lot of physical help. When in-between two fixed points – one solid object to another – I wrap both hands around a helpful arm. I'm stabilized by others and move in ways I've witnessed with the very old. The most affecting help I receive is from male friends of mine. So that we might be sitting and chatting as physical peers, but then we need to move and I become someone vulnerable, who needs their help.

As I take hold of their wrist, I'm struck by how solid it is. It might sag momentarily with my weight but then steadies and I know, or can feel, that further up this lever it's the fibres in a bicep that have shortened to steady this arm in this moment. I know this mechanism. I'm familiar with it. And I can feel, through my frail body, what I've lost. I remember it – not as an old man remembers his younger body – but from eighteen months ago; from being alongside this person who now supports me. And how I envy their body! I want it for myself.

But something else is present that feels less like this grieving for my body. Beyond the envy and the shock and sadness, is the gratitude for being helped. How can I not feel this? It's the bodily acknowledgement that what I really need in these helpless last months of my life is a father. So I can feel myself leaning into this help and feeling comfort. That's part of what's happening physically in these moments, absorbing what this feels like, this exchange, through my body – letting go and giving in to it. Wanting and needing it.

*

When Jimmy returns from nursery, I see him padding along the corridor towards me.

'Jimmy cool!' he says, and then comes to a stop in front of me.

'Ah! You've been to Jimmy school?' I ask.

'Yep,' he replies, exhaling with pleasure. 'Girls,' he then adds.

'There were girls at Jimmy school?' I ask.

'Girls!' he confirms.

'Girls? Really?'

'Yep, tractors,' he replies.

These are the biggest, most complex conversations in my life. I may talk about love and death and grief with others but nothing this profound.

'Girls and tractors?'

'Yep!' he was delighted to confirm.

'Were there? Really? That's really great! Girls and tractors at Jimmy school.'

'Me Jimmy school.'

'I know! Jimmy school sounds amazing.'

'Dinner,' he says.

'Dinner?' I ask.

He shakes his head.

'No,' he says, 'girls!'

'Dinner and girls?' I ask.

He seems startled by my reply, as if questioning how I could know this.

'Yep!'

'That sounds amazing, Jimmy!'

'Tractors.'

'Tractors?' I ask.

'And dinner,' he says, 'and girls.'

Though my tongue and vocal cords are now affected by this disease, my lips, cheeks and the muscles around the eyes and the bridge of the nose are not. So that even though I now slur, in my conversations with Jimmy, this is of less significance. With Jimmy, the communication is more bodily; it's joyous and all-consuming. If I could engage Jimmy like this for hours, I would.

I've been managing the slurring (known as dysarthria) by placing greater care and effort when enunciating multi-syllable words. A word like *elasticity* would require a long run-up and a mouthful of effort. One of the markers is with Gill or Tom – and the frequency of recent occasions on which they have had to ask me to repeat myself. At this stage, I'm able to come back with renewed energy and repeat myself, like a second attempt at vaulting a fence. It's trickier if it's noisier or busier in the house. This is when voices become more agile and melodies overlap and, when there's laughter, it's like being heard over the spin cycle of the washing machine.

At a certain point, I'll leave the group, trailing the whine of the motor from my electric wheelchair. And then someone might come to chat with me in my bedroom, knowing how much more manageable this is for me.

Over the last five years I've become more relaxed in company. It's been a gradual change and it's hard to know what to attribute this to. But I've travelled from moderate avoidance of social situations to, on occasions, craving them. So I suppose I've come closer to people and now I'm retreating back. But not as the same person. I listen to laughter and observe group behaviour, recognizing how much I would like to be part of that, but it's not a hard loss to adjust to. Other losses feel irreplaceable, but not this one. I take myself away and listen to the sound of something I was once part of. It's sad, of course, but it's also one of those changes that I'm able to regard as simply different. I've had my conversations in life; I don't absolutely need any more of them. Perhaps if I wasn't writing, I couldn't accept this; but I do.

*

I'm at my most disorientated watching Gill put shoes and socks on for me. I'm looking down at the unfamiliar view of the top of her head. Gill doesn't know this is what I see; that I am paying attention to her in this way. She feels so real to me. I'm looking at the lines of hair pulled back over her crown and thinking that I've never had the chance to see so much of her hair. Viewed from above, her head bowed and on one knee, her body takes a servile form. But I'm also looking down as a child looks down at his mother. I can't do this for myself any more. At what age did I learn to do my laces up? How long since I was here? It feels both new and rich with familiarity.

Tom can dress himself, but Jimmy and I wait our turn to have our shoes and socks put on. I've become the third child, meeting my sons going in opposite directions. And then I watch her get to me. Her husband. Her lover. How patient and efficient she is. She knows just where to pull the lace. I feel her strength, the economical movement of her hands, the drawing taut of fibres, the contraction of leather around my foot. And she is done.

At other times I wait and wait and that's about as peaceful as it gets. For some lunch. For something that I've dropped. Or sitting on the edge of the bed, naked from the waist down, with my pants and trousers around my ankles. I've got this far but lack the strength to pull them up. Gill is darting here and there and I just wait. I've found it easier than I thought, waiting. What else can I do? It's in these moments that the room seems quiet and everything is still. I've waited all my life to know this peace. To know that I am nothing more than this body.

Some segment of imagination thinks about the time to come. The thought of myself when I have lost it all. When the body is just weight. When all that's left is what's inside, still processing, still thinking. And what I can communicate now, to those I love, that it will be OK.

The Woman Who Lived
in a Shoe

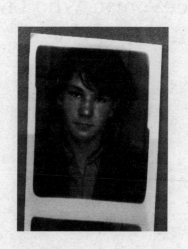

One of my aunts had been married to an Earl and they had children together. I never really knew this aunt or saw much of my cousins, who were quite a bit older than me.

But when I was around twelve or so I started considering whether I might also be nobility. I think I asked around for answers but didn't find any of the negative responses particularly helpful, even though cousins and aunts sounded like close family to me. I was startled to realize that everyone was quite old-fashioned and rules-based about these things. I tried adding *Earl* on to the front of one of my school exercise books, and even though it wasn't on the actual dotted lines where my name was supposed to go, and was sort of tagged on, I still thought it looked quite good. I started using my title here and there, but it all felt a little understated. I didn't want to make a tremendous fuss of my lineage, and I never expected anyone to use the title with my full name, but I did think it reasonable to expect that *Earl* might at least stick as some kind of nickname. I think the problem was, by this stage, *Hammondeggs* was just too well established.

At around this time I was in the habit of cycling over to visit one of the girls at school on Saturday mornings so that I could talk to her while she mucked out her horse. She was one of the kinder children at my school and I think she was sympathetic towards me. She seemed very strong and beautiful to me, with deep brown eyes and abundant dark wavy hair, and didn't seem to mind me chatting to her as she shovelled horse shit from her barn. I had probably talked to her about the frustrating lack of respect for my ancestry because I remember her putting down the shovel and coming over to talk to me. I was balanced on my bike because I never quite committed to being there, but she pulled herself up on to a low wall and seemed very serious and beautiful as she asked me why I wasn't happy being called Joe. It was a difficult question to answer and I don't think I really wanted to. It was clear to me that she wouldn't be calling me Earl and I didn't want to come straight out and ask for that because I don't think she would have agreed.

*

Even though I was quite taken with her, it was another year or so before it occurred to me that I might try being flirtatious or expressing interest in girls. Some of the other ways that I had been trying to feel better about myself always seemed to deliver limited results. I began to see that other things were going on around me with my peers and it seemed appropriate to set myself on this course of action. It wasn't driven by anything I actually felt – more by the sense of what I felt was appropriate at this stage in my life. I couldn't detect any feelings or sensations that might have been helpful in this enterprise; in the same way that you might not be able to connect your tuner to a signal because the batteries have been removed. My reference points remained those two-dimensional forms acquired when I found the stash of porn at my father's house. I was aware of what I thought intimacy looked like but not what it was. Desire was a bit like a project with a scrapbook and some glue and scissors. It makes me wonder if anyone ever took the time to make such a craft project with porn and how such a thing wouldn't be possible in the digital age. It wouldn't be a very healthy thing to do and I know I thought about the images far too much and that I hadn't really moved on in my life. I was a boy huddled over my transistor radio, fiddling with the dial, when I might have been better trying to hum a tune to myself.

I developed an increasing tendency to place myself in situations for which I was completely unprepared. I'd tried this at the age of six and, as time went on, I don't think I became any less confused. The first real occasion was in France when I was fourteen. I went with my French exchange partner and his friends to the woods, where an extremely tall, extremely confident girl waved a condom in my face as she gestured towards a small clump of trees. I followed her but, as we approached the trees, I found myself increasingly regretting the interested and experienced impression I had been trying to convey to her. I hadn't expected the situation with her to be real. Entering the soft, leafy enclosure, she knelt and, with the hand that wasn't holding the condom, pulled at my elbow to follow her downwards. At this point, I took an interest in one of the trees and, moving towards it, started scratching away at the bark with my fingernail. She called over to me and I decided it would be appropriate to feign a lack of understanding by deploying a language barrier and, after a moment, she gave a shrug, a grunt of irritation, then got up and returned to the group.

I'd like to remember this encounter in a wood in Brittany as the last moment of its kind, but instead I have to accept that I was made entirely out of wax and that, despite all the evidence this moment afforded me,

I left this woodland enclosure having moulded myself into the appearance of a functioning sexual person. I didn't stop to recognize that I lacked any kind of substance to support this. Something historic in me always felt compelled to try again, even though it was never going to work, and would be like expecting a hovercraft to hover without air, or that it might be possible to enjoy a good night's sleep on a waterbed without any water. Throughout all these years of my young life I did nothing but subject myself to experiences I never understood – as if I were a tulip in a boxing ring; a flower or a blade of grass that thinks it is another thing. Mown down or blown down and completely out of place.

*

At twenty-one, Catherine was a year older than me, and I was impressed that she owned her own flat. It didn't occur to me that she had acquired her home as the result of a personal tragedy – I just thought it was quite amazing for a person of our age. I was impressed by her French Korean heritage – and almost everything else about her – so that I didn't particularly register that she had recently lost her father and that, in a kind of way, she had lost her mother too. She was a lot brighter than anyone I had ever spent time with and this seemed to matter to me. She had needed to be independent in her life and had recently turned down the offer of a place at Cambridge University. I think I was taken with the confidence of her decision-making and resolved to do everything I could to be liked by her.

I remember that she was bothered by a nervous twitch in her eye and would spend large amounts of time using her hand as a pirate's patch. But she would always make me laugh and I don't think I ever recognized that she was feeling the loss of her father – or how it must have felt that her mother had decided to live abroad. I'm filling this memory in behind me because I wasn't attuned in that way – just as I can only now recall that the pitch of Catherine's voice heightened when she referred to any of these details and that her body – her eye and vocal cords – was flickering and vibrating and communicating her painful story. But despite this sadness, she cared for me and worried that I was squandering my life and had no plans for anything really. She knew more than me, had a greater hold on what was important, and the tender, enquiring intimacy of the way she discussed my future with me is one of the reasons I can recall her so vividly.

For several weeks, we just existed and floated or orbited together, in and out of the bookshop where we worked, along the streets of Oxford, or in cafés or sitting on a wall somewhere – and we'd always end up at her place, just listening to music and talking. And this felt like a separate existence to anything that had gone before – as if I had stepped out of something and into another something and had zipped up the opening behind me. I suppose she was *outside* and maybe that was it – not connected to anything. I think I liked that about her. And that she was ephemeral – that she had bought a plane ticket to the other side of the world and would be gone within eight weeks. She was so impressive to me and I probably tried less because of that. Maybe I felt I didn't need to try because I admired her so much and she wanted to be with me. There must have been a reason in all of this – in the details of who she was that can explain why I clung to her and why my experience with her was unlike anything that had gone before.

It happened slowly and almost imperceptibly – after days and weeks of talking and walking and laughing, about anything. This life and relationship had its own gentle pace. I think I just relaxed and slipped into being with her and it didn't feel like I was trying any more. I was just there and I don't remember that I worried much, which was strange for me, so that when our bodies gently came together, it wasn't much – or wasn't too much – as it always had been before. I don't remember even being surprised, as if I'd always been this way.

Because now it seems remarkable to me – or even something like a miracle – but at the time, I think I probably forgot that my body had ever been that different in this situation. And nothing was adept or confident about our physical relationship; just tentative and careful. It wasn't something big – just something on the map that we had shared. It wasn't everything about that time – just part of that time – and this sense of balance was something I had never previously understood. So we carried on with our days and nights together – talking and drifting and laughing and listening to music. We were intimate together and cared about each other and then she left to spend six months travelling in Korea.

*

In writing this book, and in recording the details of the difficult experiences from my early life, I also want to record details of the people who have helped me. It's no surprise to me that every religion of any kind that's ever existed has developed a belief in the spirits that surround us in our lives. It seems to me that souls are always transmigrating and transmogrifying willynilly and have absolutely no interest in delaying their departure for the formality and finality of death. Such promiscuity is essential because, where spirits exist, there upon a muddy bank also sits a long line of toads. So there are two presences in life: there are the spirits that are all around us and there are the stinky, warty, stolid toads lined up in opposition.

I am as aware of the spirits as I am of the toads. And having already written of the toads, it's a pleasure and a necessity to write about the spirits too. And just as the toads never really leave, even if you kick them, neither do the spirits. Some people might choose to explain these presences as a product of what adheres from life's good and bad experiences, but that does nothing to explain the stink of a toad or the oily mess it leaves behind. Whilst memory of that time with Catherine fades a little, and despite the way I let her down in the end, and even though I turned away from something so precious, and even tried to deny that it ever existed, despite all of this, the wing-shaped presence from that time in my life still flits around my ears and is about as solid as a house-brick.

It's therefore obvious that I will never really die; not *really* die. And that the spirits in my life – those I am now starting to tell you about – are already forming with my own in some splendid fairy commotion, not unlike the spectacle of a crowded outdoor swimming pool in summer, and that I will be a spirit completely free from my body, and that I will always be and that I will never leave Gill's side, or Tom's, or Jimmy's, for as long as they need me. This strikes me as something so clear and unquestionable that it hardly needs saying.

*

When the letters started arriving they took the form of opened-up paper bags from Korean fast-food restaurants, ornately covered on both sides with criss-crossing stories and messages and annotations. The first of the letters startled me because, in a way that now seems incomprehensible, I hadn't been expecting to hear from Catherine again.

I laid its geometric presence out flat in front of me and naively examined the artefact for evidence of what this meant. Very little had been discussed on the way up the escalators to the departure terminal or in those moments when I lay on her bed watching Catherine place folded items into her suitcase. But over a period of months the letters kept coming, emblazoned with Korean promises of tasty food – and funny stories and doodles – and no sense at all of something having ended. And at the foot of her very final letter was a flight number.

I kept a few of the belongings that she had discarded in the process of packing, but these were never items I thought to use. I just liked their familiar fragrance, and I laid them out on the little table near my bed. There was a small black knapsack and a collection of pens in a blue fabric pencil case. I also held on to her potted palm, and I was unusually diligent in watering it and keeping its leaves free from dust. But with the letters themselves, I don't know where I kept them – amongst a pile of papers perhaps, or tucked away in a drawer somewhere, as items of lesser significance.

When Catherine flew in, I was at the airport, but I wondered if this had occurred by accident, or whether I was there to pick up someone completely different. With the sorry way I was ambling through the concourse, it seemed most plausible that I was a refugee from somewhere, without the means for onward or return travel. By some freak chance, I happened to be standing at the arrivals gate at exactly the time Catherine emerged. She looked tired as she glanced along a line of people leaning into a chrome rail, but when she finally picked me out from the grey faces of those hanging back, there was enormous warmth in her smile. On reflection, a genuine smile, when a person's *really* tired, can be something quite beautiful. I'm talking about that point of tiredness when someone is so exhausted it takes profound pleasure for a smile to emerge. And then it's something slow and languid and lasting.

I don't think I appreciated this beauty at the time. I may well have pointed at my chest, miming the words

'Who, me?' And then I might have glanced around, hoping that someone else might have been the recipient.

In all the years leading up to this moment, I encountered a lot of bemusement, and often some level of self-questioning, from those I had tried to convince, through sleight of hand, that I possessed some kind of prowess. Occasionally, I encountered relief. There had been grunts of annoyance, as with that first time in a French wood. But if I half remember these reactions as somewhat watery two-dimensional images, from Catherine's face, over the next few months, I harvested a deep, shimmering palette of three-dimensional disappointment and sadness.

Catherine stuck with my stultifying presence for a while, before realizing that, all this time, I had been bent double, walking backwards along our path, attempting to rub and scrub out all traces of the troubling closeness we had once shared.

The expression of Catherine's that I remember most was from the last occasion that we saw each other, on some nondescript central London street. I remember this because, if there had been any expressions of contempt from her during this period, they had long since been replaced by a kind of fatigue and tedium. Quite understandably, she'd had enough and, in a very sad and straightforward way, said goodbye and disappeared through the ticket barrier of an Underground station.

*

I sat inside my car in the rain and ate fried chicken with the windscreen wipers on. I think a letter came from the bookshop telling me that, due to prolonged absenteeism, I was no longer an employee, and I stuffed it inside the glove compartment. I imagine this was autumn and that the leaves fell from the trees for over a year and that they never seemed to stop. I walked down roads and when I got to the end I crossed back over and walked back again. I had various temping jobs in warehouses, moving boxes from one end of a large building to another, or taking things out of boxes, or putting them back in again. And in this time, most of the people I knew moved away in different kinds of ways, and I tended to walk around or drive around on my own.

I increasingly preferred staying in my car or remaining at home because of the inconvenient ways in which my body started leaking sadness at a bus stop or when paying for something at the checkout. And I remember having a problem with blushing, so that it was hard to buy stamps at the post office or pay in a cheque at the bank. There seemed to be so much wrong with my body, and I was happy to tell the doctor what kinds of tests he might commission, but once I'd started offering him my different theories and opinions, it was very hard to stop. To enable his understanding, I thought it best to keep coming back, and I was always so positive during these appointments. I think I smiled a lot and had really good manners – always stopping to check that he understood what I was explaining to him – and it was only afterwards, in the street, that I'd pinch my cheeks to try and stem what was coming. And with the heat from my face it would feel like grease rather than tears and I'd sit at the outside trestle table of the pub next door, lowering my head between my knees and making dark little patterns on the tarmac.

*

In writing about spirits, I suppose I am acknowledging that there isn't a person who ever existed who hasn't, in some way, by the end of their life – particularly towards the end of their life – composed or reflected upon the architecture of their very own religion. And when I think about what this is, I have in mind those moments when Tom comes to me in my wheelchair or my hospital bed and I will hold out my good left hand, palm upwards, and then he will gently rest his palm down on mine. And what exists there between us is just the smoothness of our skin and the warmth we have created. And then

Tom will ask me something, like where the Sellotape is; or he will tell me that dinner is almost ready or that the cardboard house he is working on now has a new roof. The question will then be addressed and answered in some form, and then he will be gone, leaving the trace of himself on my upturned palm.

I've found different aspects of physical life very difficult and there is something of a great personal narrative climaxing in what is now happening to my body. But I have felt that love is a physical act – as it is in these exchanges with my son. At different times it is the physicality of love that has struck me and how strong the body is when it feels love for someone; and how weak when it doesn't.

When I was young, there was one glorious adult in my life who, in this physical respect, was completely apart from all the other toads lined up there on the muddy bank. Jean was a tall and slightly gangly friend of my mum's, with extremely long, straight dark hair and a conspicuous mole on the waxy brown surface of her right cheek. She always seemed so strong and, for all the majesty she held for me, this social worker from north London might as well have been chief of the Apaches or an Egyptian queen.

She smoked a lot and laughed a lot and offered me the permanent impression that what she wanted was to laugh about the situation she and I were in. And with this single motivation: that both of us must share in the hysterics of the moment. Her eyes always prefigured her laughter and, when this laughter came, it rippled in her face like chain reactions prior to eruption. And then it felt like she and I were holding hands, feeling each of these vibrations. Hers was a seismic compressed laughter – bubbling and jostling behind her pursed lips. But when it came, when the lips gave way, the sound it created was informed by the texture of her smoking. It was a vast spillage of a laugh. A wheeze and a wobble and a scream that would take my legs from under me and wash me away to a place, with this woman.

Though slender, she was a physical presence, with power in her hands. She would grab me and squeeze me and, in those moments, I melted through her skin and just rested there for all the time I needed. I saw her very little – perhaps once or twice a year – but, when I did, all my preoccupations dropped away like petals in October. I didn't have to dance or be a thing or guess the direction of the wind. She looked at me as if she already knew everything there was to know. She knew it all without me saying – as if I ever could – and whirled me around and pulled me to her chest and kept me there and filled me up until it was time for her to leave.

*

The consulting room was a wooden shed set back within the garden of a large house on the affluent northern side of the city. I'd enter a tiny reception area at the front of this garden shed and, after a few moments, the internal door would open and another client might exit; at other times it would just be her and she would gesture for me to come inside. I would lie down on what was a narrow, flat bed, with a pillow under my head, with the woman seated out of view, just behind me.

Next to my feet there was a table with a small potted plant and a box of tissues. If I arched my neck upwards I could see the very simple light fitting immediately above my head. Apart from these features, within a field of vision that took in perhaps sixty per cent of the room, there was one slightly more interesting item that I spent the next six years, and up to four times a week, examining and trying to understand. On the right-hand wall, next to a window, was a small, framed reproduction of a nineteenth-century painting in which a woman kneels in the furrow of a freshly tilled field, presumably planting seed. Just behind and to the left, her very young child sits on the hem of his mother's dress playing in the earth.

I was now twenty-one and for the first four years I said very little and winced at the few things I did say. I became adept at memorizing my dreams because it meant I didn't have to think of anything to say. It had been suggested that the opportunity to bring thoughts and feelings to these appointments might enable me to function more effectively in my relationships but, instead, the opposite became true. I moved into a bed-sit so that I could live on my own and my contact with friends and family declined. My life consisted of a clerical job in a large office and extended lunchtime appointments at the garden shed.

Throughout these four years I held a very low opinion of the woman who sat behind me at my appointments. Though I could have stopped at any point, I assailed her with a continual list of her many and obvious faults, mainly relating to her incompetence and lack of professionalism, along with the preposterous, ridiculous nature of almost everything she said. I consistently questioned her credentials and even told her she was unbearably ugly. She had a large house with evidence of family life and perhaps my main gripe was that she couldn't possibly care for me, with all these children of her own and other clients to look after. Her faults seemed so obvious to me and I came to realize that her difficulties had been widely known for some time:

> There was an old woman who lived in a shoe.
> She had so many children, she didn't know what to do.

Despite her being relatively young, this was so clearly the woman in question, and such a perfectly concise indictment of her crimes, but I lacked the confidence to report her to the appropriate prosecuting body. So I continued like this, month after month, year after year. It was a vast expanse of time that passed – a period of time in which I could reasonably have qualified in a number of quite advanced professions, or mastered several musical instruments; I could have built a large house for myself with my own garden shed or, a little more adventurously, trekked across a continent or two. But instead of considering these possibilities I maintained a clerical job with a hole-punch and a lever arch file and, despite my frustrations and suspicions, continued to attend my appointments inside the garden shed.

*

By the fifth year I was living in a bedsit at the top of a vast Victorian town house divided into twenty or so other bedsits. And by this time, it could almost have been something Alexandre Dumas might have written – an epic love story, with religious overtones, about a man in a tower wearing an iron mask; whereas I was a boy in a bedsit with the curtains closed, masturbating into a tissue twice a day. In fact, this had been my third or fourth such room, but I liked the anonymity this one provided, and also the advantage of the single bathroom I shared with a resident who was never at home. I stored food in my room to avoid using communal kitchen cupboards and timed my runs to the kitchen fridge to avoid other residents. On weekends, and particularly religious holidays, I was especially careful to manage my provisions in such a way that I could remain completely out of view. On the previous Christmas I had been caught with my head in the fridge by a joyous Spanish couple who vigorously persuaded me to share their lunch with them but who then, after prolonged exposure to my company, lost so much blood to their faces and vital organs that I was able to retreat carefully away, thirty minutes or so later, without the three of us even needing to say a word to each other – as if I had walked backwards out of a still photo.

During the long hours I spent in that room I watched a lot of television. On Saturdays, a reliable segment of the middle of the day would be consumed by the build-up to the 3 p.m. football kick-offs and the subsequent post-match analysis. It was fortuitous that, at about this time, Channel 4 started broadcasting live Italian football on Sundays and this offered the ideal equivalent match-day experience. Both days of the weekend I used this central sporting chunk as a kind of tent pole to my waking hours and, either side of this, I managed the preparation and consumption of breakfast, lunch and dinner – laid out on a tray upon my lap. It was an arrangement that enabled each day to pass without too many empty intervals and, before long, I would be through to the engulfing commitment of my clerical job. And weeks would pass like this and months turned into years – Monday through to Sunday, New Year through to Christmas.

*

Recalling this despair and emptiness, it's of little surprise that God appeared to me in one very specific moment, when I was parked up in an old blue Saab 900 by a river, and spoke to me with quite the clarity that he did. He did so in the summer gap between the fifth and sixth year of my appointments inside the garden shed. When this moment took place, I was sitting in my stationary vehicle on the edge of a field, leaking oil from an unfixable engine gasket. I had the driver's side door open and was seated on the passenger side, set to full recline, so that I was able to put my feet on the dashboard and lie back reading my book, with all four windows wound down, so that the early-evening air cooled my skin as it went racing by.

It was in this year that I had moved on from reading spy novels and had worked my way through most of George Eliot and a lot of Dickens, so that by the summer I was mainly concentrating on translations of Dostoevsky. And this was my reading material in that moment when God spoke to me through the rusting petrol-blue bodywork of my car, by the side of the river. Specifically, it was *The Brothers Karamazov* – a tale of three brothers born to a wanton father. I think I may have felt this moment moving closer and I had parked up in this spot between two footpaths so that I could finish this book in a setting other than my bedsit. In that sense, it could be said that I was looking for something, or that it had been building, so that I had perhaps selected this very special location in preparation for the approach I knew was coming.

I should say that the literary aspect to all of this didn't occur in isolation. During the fifth year of appointments with the woman in the garden shed, I had started to relax a little more. I began to notice a few details about the voice that existed behind me and one of these details was an occasional tendency to relate one of her observations to a literary reference or quotation. I was able to infer that, despite living in a shoe and having vast numbers of children to look after, she still managed to find a bit of time in her day to read. I had been an early reader, but when the difficulties took root in my childhood everything fell away and I left school at sixteen with very little interest in books or anything else.

So there had been some changes over the course of about a year that led up to this moment in my car with this book – perhaps a kind of loosening of something that had become impacted. And when it happened I would describe it as a penetrating warmth and something ligamental that was softening and lengthening. My body felt less tight and this was almost instantaneous. I can't remember but I imagine, in that moment, I would have needed to adjust my heels on the dashboard to accommodate this. It was also the accelerated sensation of being noticed in a very direct kind of way, which was both unsettling and comforting at the same time. It wasn't possible to disentangle all these feelings and, at this initial stage, I felt no impulse or awareness that I might actually talk with this sudden presence in my life. It was enough, with the seat reclined and my feet up on the veneered black dashboard, just to notice the resistance easing in my body, like the depth change that wood or metal vessels undergo when coming to the surface – the tiny creaks and pops and hisses of a body expanding to its natural state.

In the weeks that followed the incident in the car, my body felt different. This change was dramatic and quite sudden; instant, in fact. I even considered the possibility that I might have become an inch or two taller, which is the way it felt. A lot of the simple mechanisms in my life felt somehow easier: walking, for example. At home in my bedsit, I enjoyed putting my lengthening strides to the test around the large Victorian building. I no longer felt it necessary to frequent the kitchen during significantly off-peak hours, such as three in the morning; in fact, as my confidence grew, there were even occasions when I chose to use the communal cooking facilities during conventional dinner times and found myself sharing the kitchen with a range of fellow housemates. We even struck up conversations and I no longer felt a pain in my forehead when someone smiled at me. It actually felt natural to smile back or even to laugh about something with another person. It meant that I could form facial expressions that were wholly new to me and which caused a slight delay in the reactions of housemates or colleagues as they examined my face for evidence of whether what they were experiencing was a good thing or an extremely worrying thing.

*

It feels like the appropriate time to tackle the question of whether God exists or not. Not whether God exists but the *question* of whether he exists. It's a question that belongs in the same category as 'Why doesn't anybody love me?' or 'Why do I never feel good enough?' A person who properly knows that God *doesn't* exist would never waste their time asking this question. To be asking whether God exists, a person must find it so hard to feel certain or confident about even the most simple things in life: to know whether the chair they are sitting on really exists or whether the kisses they receive in life were ever really meant.

It's only possible to *luxuriate* in the question of whether God exists or not. So that if your home is threatened by mortar shells or if you live in a time of famine and must notice the bloating in your children's bellies, you either know God exists or know that he doesn't. When I was desperate and leaking sadness in my life it was also very clear to me. And now that I'm leaving my wife with a two-year-old and a six-year-old, with no money, and with no family who can safely look after them if something happens to Gill, I don't feel comfortable enough to question God. Everything I love is teetering high up and out of reach. There is nothing I can do but know God, as I assume everyone finally does, when these moments come.

*

I apologized to the woman in the garden shed for comments in which I had compared her to a series of farmyard animals; in fact, she bore a much closer resemblance to a female TV presenter and panel-show host who was particularly popular at that time. I also apologized for saying insulting things about her family – something that I then felt extremely ashamed about and always have. I must have made these comments over a year before, but I had just returned after the long summer break and it was the first occasion when an apology had even occurred to me. I also thought about how boring and unpleasant that five-year period must have been for her and how much of her professional time I had taken up. Five years I had spent inside this tiny space, staring up at the light fitting, with its pot plant and its box of tissues and its smell of carpet and pine – and I think, on that first appointment after the summer, I looked around as if this had been my very first time in this tiny room. Or that I had taken my iron mask off and had looked around to find myself waist deep in five years' worth of used paper tissues.

I'd been wanting to tell the woman in the garden shed about God – the God who appears in cars on the edges of rivers in summer – but in the way that a child might come home from school and want to show the model of the universe he made from string and ping-pong balls. And I think the respect and care she took with my creation is something that has continued to make all the difference to me. I think of that moment on that bed, with her voice knowing and understanding me completely, as being the most important in my life; and that without it, very little would have been possible.

I spent another year in the garden shed but had already started making up for my lack of qualifications by attending evening classes, so that a year or two later I enrolled at university in another part of the country. I don't think my experience inside the garden shed enabled a huge amount to change in my life, but it was enough. I sold my old blue Saab 900 for scrap and, after that, God was never quite as intimate or loud as he had been before. But he'd made himself known and the memory of that remained important for me. Of most significance was that I had spent this time in a room with someone. It was as simple and as hard as that.

Gill

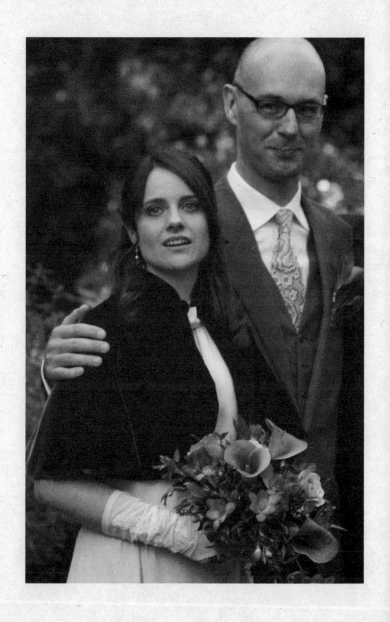

Near where the M40 slices through the Chilterns at High Wycombe or Beaconsfield, there's a piece of graffiti spelling out *Why do I still do this every day?* in wonky fridge-magnet capital letters, along a stretch of concrete sidings a hundred yards or so from the road, high up on a grassy bank. Gill and I were looking at it from the coach on the way to London and we were talking about our futures and what we imagined for them. We'd been together a year or so by then and the conversation was about how difficult it would be for us because we were two wounded figures. We knew it about each other – that we had been ill, at times, in our lives; and frightened.

It had been a more serious fifteen-mile stretch of motorway than the initial section of the A40 heading out of Oxford. I don't know why it changed or why certain things came up. We imagined being older together. We imagined being a mum and dad. It felt like pulling down the small table from the seat in front and placing something on it from a pocket, just to take a look.

And my perspective now, in remembering that moment, is from above, looking down at us in that traffic: these two figures side by side at the back of a coach, talking and wondering and doubting. I think about the children's book, *The Borrowers*, about a tiny family, each a few inches tall, who live in the walls and under the floors of a country house. They manage by borrowing and adapting to make a home for themselves, so that a borrowed thimble becomes a bucket, or a cotton reel becomes a chair. I think we were such little people – we didn't come from anywhere. We shared this: that we didn't belong.

We were on that bus imagining a life together that we didn't understand, on a coach going along that stretch of the M40 just prior to the junction with the M25; before London starts building up: looking out through the window at the sidings and the graffiti and knowing it was both possible and unlikely. And we would have felt scared, wondering if it would be us together a year or so further on, still imagining and believing in something for ourselves, or whether we would be on our own again: two figures on a coach on the motorway talking and thinking and being together; not knowing, really, what this was.

And yet we lived together, travelled together, worked things out together and bought a house together; we had children together. But always as composites of things that adults should already have understood. So many aspects of life we pieced together from discarded egg boxes and the cardboard from used breakfast cereals. We licked them and stuck them together and, over the years, we pieced all this together with Sellotape and decked our lives out with silver foil. Nothing was already there and we made this together into something that worked as well as anything ever could. Nothing real was given. We have been Styrofoam artists with the treasure from a wheelie bin that we pushed out on to the street on Friday mornings. And all these years later, something whole has been pieced together from these scraps of milk-bottle tops and used loo roll, so that everything has been created from something else. And at a certain moment the sea appeared and what we had made proved as solid as anything sleek and uniform or plastic that floated by. And I wonder what will happen to it and whether it will still exist in the future. What will it be? What will it be worth at the salvage yard or to anybody else? This tattery thing that I made with someone else.

*

At almost a foot taller than Gill, I knew the place on my chest where the left side of her face came to rest when something felt overwhelming. The strap of Gill's bra would push into the palm on my right hand and, with my fingertips, I could feel several of the ribs at the back of her chest. And when her body moved it was like a series of extremely rapid shrugs, and the tip of my chin would carefully touch down on the crown of her head so that I could move more effectively to her rhythm in these moments.

Until a year ago, I had fallen a long way behind Gill. If your life is not quite functioning, as mine wasn't, it's not obvious what you should cry about and so you might cry about a crisp packet or a bus ticket, if anything at all, and never really know why. So in this moment with Gill I might as well have had two hands flat on the sides of a food processor, or both clasped around the handles of a powerful lawnmower. These were largely cerebral embraces and I was doing little more than holding on but, as the movement in Gill's chest cavity and diaphragm subsided, she would pull back and I would see her more clearly. The tips of her cheeks would appear pink and swollen and drenched, with the residue of her left eye socket as a neatly printed triangle of moisture on my T-shirt and a tightrope of salty mucous still connecting us.

Sometimes I would feel frustrated because perhaps I was browning some onions in a pan or was on the way to the bathroom to trim my nose hair. Or perhaps it had been one of several episodes in which Gill had felt sad or overwhelmed over a period of a few days and I wanted it to end, so that my inert body wouldn't need a further reminder of this warmth and this movement.

I wonder if Gill now observes the way *my* face changes: the way I cry by trying to connect the tips of my cheeks to the bridge of my nose and pulling down my bottom lip into an impossible V. I think this must be strange – to be next to my body when it is finally working and responding to loss in this way, and wishing there was more time for the two of us to share this knowledge: that we could go crying together, perhaps to different places around the world, in the same way that we go walking together. We could finally go crying together to Japan or sobbing to the Outer Hebrides, just like we'd planned.

Years go by and the shapes you make with another person become moulded into who you are together: shapes in bed together or on a sofa or standing. And after many years together, it might be easier not to love, or to find somebody else to love, than to change the little indents or the handholds that time has smoothed so perfectly. The places now available to me are all such solo locations: in my wheelchair or recliner or in my hospital bed. I might be in a gully or high up on a cliff. What must it feel like in that moment when Gill is overwhelmed and, where my giant legs once stood, the little engine of my wheelchair spins around and around? It's like the clay or plasticine has hardened and there's nothing but edges and metal legs or armrests in the way. And we message our distress with walkie-talkies or leave paper notes with little droplets for each other; until that moment near the fridge – two weeks ago – next to a fallen cube of Lego, when her hip slipped in below my arm and the left side of my face softened in below her breasts. Not quite leaving dark prints from my eye socket; just feeling that I wanted to be inside here with all of my face and how soft and warm this body is.

And now I have this other opportunity, when I have to wake Gill in the middle of the night to help me up. I have started sleeping in a hospital style bed, alongside the larger one we used to share. It has a button to lift my head and torso, but it's never quite enough when I'm limp and sleepy. So Gill comes around to be by my side, reaching in and clasping her hands behind my back, pulling me upright. And there I am again, dropping sweetly into her softness and her strength – slumped and mumbling, and no longer cerebral.

*

Gill's body works really well. She doesn't see it this way – she feels her body to be stretched and dragged by everything that is happening – but when I drop a fork or my phone or my water bottle on the floor, the movement made as she picks it up reminds me of the way a golfer collects their ball from the hole after a successful putt or the way a flamingo smoothly lowers its bill into the water to collect a fish. I suppose I now observe these efficient bodily mechanisms more acutely than before.

I say thank you a lot to Gill. It must be thousands of times a day and I mean it so much. It's not manners; I don't employ any manners with Gill. I probably used to, but these days it's just gratitude that comes tumbling out of me for all the things she now has to do for me. That's a nice feeling to have so much of.

The differences between our bodies does separate us; the difference between air and stone. Babies must feel lonely, with so much movement circling them, before they work out how good things really are. I tend to remain in one place and Gill is so much more mobile. I can hear a lot of what she's doing. I can hear the bin lid or the front door or a pan being dragged from a cupboard. And I'm following her movements around the house and the footsteps in the hallway that I always hope will bring her to me.

*

It was October and we'd known each other a month. We were walking down the high street holding hands when I stopped and pointed at the coat in the window. Gill turned to look but only in its general direction, with her head moving in a more panoramic mode than I would have expected. This was a small boutique shop and the coat was on display at the very front. Everything else was folded or draped but the coat was on a stand, so that it could be seen full length by everyone who glanced in its direction.

I jabbed my finger coatwards but could see Gill's eyes chase her smile around her face, like one of those small handheld toys where you have to get several tiny silver balls to stay in place at the same time. I stood back with Gill on the pavement and we stood with our arms touching, facing the coat together, with people streaming by. There it was: a conspicuous black parka-style winter coat with a silver faux-fur hood and I wondered why she couldn't see it. I tried to make the suggestion more intimately – how she mentioned she was cold without a winter coat. And I think in this moment my hands were making tumbling and pointing gestures, as if I were participating in a collective dance move, on a school gym floor under coloured lights. But really, it was the feeling of being in a foreign city with a phrase book and the warmth of the embarrassment from someone so amiable and forgiving.

Five years later we owned our own flat and fitted a new floor and a fireplace, but for Gill it all went back to the coat, and also the mushroom risotto I made when we arrived at my place. She had watched me with such excitement, as I put butter and cheese into the pan, and smiled so much that our teeth clashed when we kissed for the first time a few moments later. I was cooking at the open end of someone else's history and I like the idea that this was some small part of why Gill fell in love with me: that I was someone who thought she might need a coat when she was cold or a meal when she was hungry.

*

Gill helps me out of bed, she puts a teabag in a cup and wraps a blanket around me, so that I can start work. It's 4 a.m. and, midway through the question 'Is that it?', she touches me softly with her palm cupped over my wrist, opens up a yawn and turns to go back to bed.

I met Gill when I had just started writing plays. She shared in the excitement of that time and we read plays together and saw plays together, until I lost my way and didn't know why I was doing it or what else I should be doing.

And now I'm sitting down in the small hours to write about this person. This person with a mind and a body who I took so long to understand and be with. Now that I have come back to writing, I'm writing about *her*, and that feels like the best of ways to end this.

Everything takes so long and is nearly gone, apart from the millions of moments still remaining.

*

There was a moment last week when I was lying in bed and heard Gill and Jimmy on the other side of the door. Something had piqued Jimmy's curiosity – some kind of container or a tool, perhaps – and he was employing one of his new 'What this?' phrases. Their voices weren't in any way muffled and I could see the shadow of their movements through the slit at the foot of the door. I could tell they were sitting there together, contemplating the identity of an object, and Gill was guiding his hand in its operation, so that the joyous sounds were of oohs and aahs, with very little explanation.

I'm writing this and thinking about what it means to be self-taught. I think it's less to do with the private nature of the learning, more that a person arrives at a point in their life when they might already expect or want themselves to know something vital but don't. The knowledge isn't formed developmentally; it's a chasm waiting to be filled.

I hear Gill with our children and I can hear the beeps of large machinery reversing; the vast sides of earth being turned up like a playing card and moved. Even though Gill is exhausted and wants to stop, I can tell she is digging into me and moving me around – turning over the chasm I've been filling in all these years and expanding into it, as she now has to, in the momentary spaces of the day and at night. She knows in her body how to do this. I hear her voice with our children and how the sounds she now makes are mine as well: that in the lonely hours, she is becoming both of us. It can't be stopped by self-doubt – it's happening anyway – even in the dark and in the rain, high up there in the cab of a vast digger. The chasm of knowledge she is filling. The power of it. Tom and Jimmy know this too.

*

Until it was destroyed by fire, Gill spent several years as a young girl living on a boat, and up to the point at which we settled to live in our London flat, none of her subsequent homes had proved in any way reliable.

We lived in our flat for fifteen years. Tom was born in its living room, and for Gill, surrounded as we were by trees and a rare London silence, ascending all these flights of stairs to the top always felt like a perch or a parapet, high up in the skies. It was safe and unexpected, like the experience of a new coat. And I know this safe, beloved home is where Gill always expected to return to: this high-up place, now out of reach to us.

Nobody who has ever felt unsafe as a child ever loses that feeling completely. And the fact that we are having to sell the flat is stirring all of this. We're miles from home but still a little fear is crumbling away, under her feet and in the plaster of the walls. It doesn't matter where we are – I see the little tremors where she walks, and all the cracks appearing in the ceiling overhead. I can see it's always there – how at night she slips between the tiny gap at the edges of our bed.

And when I have any dreams for Gill and Tom and Jimmy, they are masonry dreams and garden dreams and room dreams, of somewhere they will one day live. I want to find this place, to build it in the night, whirring around foundations in my chair, with a trowel in my good hand and a mortar board on my lap.

*

I remember that we were crossing over from Crystal Palace Park to Westow Hill and I was expressing frustration with my writing career, a subject that I was carrying around with me, even on a walk in the park. We were standing at the traffic lights and Gill was walking ahead as she said, without looking at me, that she wasn't interested. The lights had turned green and I missed my step and then I shuffled forward to catch her up.

I could write this chapter as a history of all the different ways Gill has waited for me or made allowances, or the many different sizes of sacrifices she made, until she didn't – like this moment, five years ago, as the lights turned green, and she wasn't going to wait any more, for anyone.

Everything gets heavier as you get older, so that you can end up as a person weighed down, wearing several hundred coats, with the pockets full of other people's pebbles. Maybe you're born with a duffel jacket draped around your shoulders; perhaps a trench coat as well.

Gill was born ten years after her siblings, into the disappointment of a failing marriage, and spent her life managing other people's expectations until this time, around five years ago, when she decided not to. At this time in her life she had decided that other people's disappointments or frustrations were not her responsibility and never had been. I noticed the telephone conversations with her family getting shorter, and how she'd always spend these calls removing several dozen overcoats, with the phone pinned between her cheek and shoulder, or how she returned discarded jackets into my arms as I stood waiting at traffic lights.

I could see that Gill was enjoying her work more and that people respected her in ways they hadn't before and that the fewer coats she wore the more people respected her and wanted to spend time with her. She had an independence that surprised me. I was both interested in it and surprised by it. And I didn't know if I would be good enough for this person or that I ever had been.

I'm glad I cared enough to be frightened in this moment and I now see it's not always the right thing to wait for those pedestrians who fail to notice that the lights at the crossing have turned green. This must be the point when marriages fail in so many different and sad little ways. And even though it was painful for me, I think I owe Gill a lot for these changes she made in her life and for the opportunity they also gave me. Because I never intended to take advantage or take for granted, but I suppose these things happen slowly or are even there at conception.

I saw the truth approaching the kerb on the other side of the road and that is all I did – I saw her, and recognized what it was, and that it was crossing the road away from me. I kept going and tried to keep up, because that's as much as I could manage at the time. I didn't turn left on my own to go down Anerley Road or Crystal Palace Parade because I didn't want to lose her;

I wanted to follow her. I think it was the excitement of it. That really was the thing – the excitement of another person.

*

I know the gods are not against Gill, even though she feels they are. There are some gods from the 1963 movie of *Jason and the Argonauts* – indolent gods in togas, with someone in the background playing the lyre – and these gods may be against her but not the other ones.

Gill took us to Portugal and she carried us back. And that's quite a thing for a parent and a carer, without a viable mother and father of their own, to be both the mind and the muscle of a family, without the feeling that it's ever possible to stop or let go.

And for someone who gave up her career for this, and then got punished with a husband who is sick and dying, and with the sky falling on her head most days, and a lot of shit and wee to clear up, I know it all seems really bad, which it is. It's probably worse than it seems, or will be. The gods may end up proving to be even more capricious, and the shit and wee even more copious, which I realize is not the most reassuring thing for me to say.

It's not necessary to be strong. I suppose people just live through things, which is what I see. And I don't even know if it will get better; it might get worse! But at some point the sun has to stream down on the carnage and make pretty patterns in the glistening pools of evaporating pee. In this moment I know Gill will feel like peace and that bits of this will feel funny enough to properly laugh at.

Mooto Nuney Disease

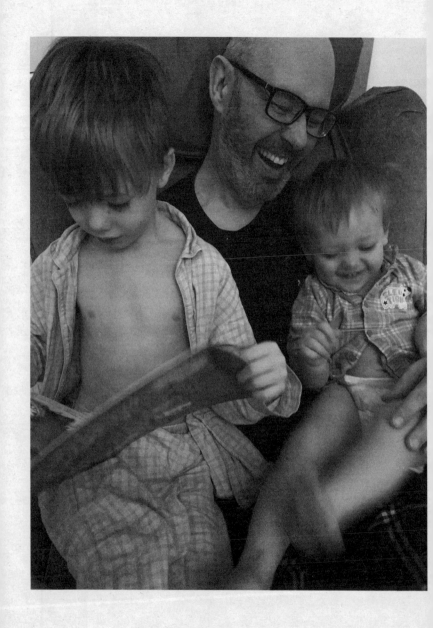

I came into the room late with my wheelchair whirring and could see that a friend was holding Tom by his ankles over the sofa. My son was making a happy version of the sound that lobsters are supposed to make when they're dropped into boiling water.

I know that one day there may be other important men in Tom and Jimmy's life and it's hard not knowing if these relationships will be OK. I just have to trust that they will be, which is another way of letting go and knowing that it's never possible to have control; not really. It's a useful kind of knowledge to have finally arrived at – to let go of something I never really had hold of.

For three years, until Tom was four, Gill worked full time as a teacher and I worked the weekends. I was at home with Tom, and so the history of our lives is closely bound together. I was a mother to my boy, and a father too. I was a kind of mother to Gill as well and I had confidence in what the three of us could be. I was the architect of our young family, and later that role became Gill's. She just couldn't be this person at the beginning. Confidence moves around and I realize now that I've had distinct periods of it in my life that began with the year of briefly knowing God in a very intimate way and is ending with the discovery of dying. Between these two was the excitement and the power I felt in the early years of writing plays, and the years that I'm reflecting on now, in which I looked after my son and our young family.

But now I'm more detached: I'm almost Scrooge returning to a life in which he never existed or Jimmy Stewart's character in *It's a Wonderful Life*. So that walking in to see a friend playing with Tom makes me feel like I'm not quite here and that I'm dreaming of a different time. It's a dream of something and is painful in a way I have begun to accept. Gill sometimes nudges Tom to acknowledge me or say goodnight to me, and there was a period a few weeks ago when he seemed resistant to this. Our lives are stressful and I think Tom was feeling a little insecure at school, so perhaps he was crowding out other relationships to get as much as possible from his mummy. This meant that days went by in which I could say something and he appeared not to hear me, or that he would walk by me as if I was invisible and I would cup my heart carefully like it was raspberry jelly.

Some time went by in this vein, and I could feel my confidence slipping, but then one morning, and I don't know why, Tom climbed up on to my bed and nestled his face into the pit of my shoulder. I didn't want to move and I think I even slowed down my breathing. Then he moved and I thought this moment was lost but he was turning to lie with his chest on mine and the side of his face pressed flat on to my sternum, so that his arms draped over the sides of my body. I continued to look at the ceiling because, most of all, I didn't want anything to change; except that I moved my hand in one gentle stroke of the back of his hair, down to the nape of his neck, and kept my hand on his shoulder blade until he got up, about twenty seconds later.

I've fallen on hard times – that's what this is – and I've become adept at extracting pleasure from less. It's the experience of poverty, and a child who might receive something frugal at Christmas but feels more joy than most. So my life as a parent can be exquisite in ways it could never be before. I know what these moments are and I hope I'm ready for them, whenever they might come.

*

Gill and Tom had formed themselves into a rolling ball of feet and hair because I had wanted the black bits from between Tom's toes to sprinkle on my scrambled eggs. But it didn't work and Tom finished the manoeuvre sitting on the back of Gill's head with a very wide grin.

Children are like ivy, the way they reach into you and wrap around you, asking questions with their bodies and finding routes through. Part of my learning that love is something physical was learnt in moments with Tom when he was young and I cared for him. I'm describing something physical that other parents know but which I discovered as if it were a hidden kingdom. So that the world could churn around and jostle and bobble uncontrollably for my young son, and I found that all this discombobulation could be stilled if we sat together and I spread my large open hand on Tom's chest and held it there whilst his heart settled those few inches away from the warmth of my palm. Or that it was sometimes necessary to twirl Tom like a baton around my neck or use him like a wheelbarrow or roll him up like sushi in a duvet. Just to be big with my arms and chest and back and let him know that this great frame of mine was moving in his life to be with him and to keep him warm and safe.

This knowledge is now locked away, as I look out at the physical world of these people I love. It won't be my children's memory of me, just an artefact glimpsed in photos and the odd film – something they will one day interpret. Disappearing like this is a way of letting go of ego and that's a calm feeling; it makes me feel like a slightly better person, in a way that I would otherwise never have achieved. I see who Tom and Jimmy are and now think more broadly about what their lives will be – the large canvas of their future welfare, with its many clean white spaces. Many of the decisions I now make, or make with Gill, are about a time that should have involved me but now won't. I like ending my life in this way, as a parent – and I like the small contribution it now makes to repairing a life that has long been insecure and, in part, vain or self-absorbed.

I'm looking over and Gill is there with her body and her face pushed down into the duvet as Tom sits smiling on top of her head. I'm watching this, knowing he's not alone and that at least one of us can remind and reassure that love is physical and real and always there for him. And my place in all of this is becoming smaller, historic and just the right size of important.

*

I was wrapped in yellow and orange blankets at the edge of the yard, shrieking like a tiny broken accordion. It's January and I only go outside once or twice a week. A lot is involved in getting me ready for outdoors and I never want to put Gill through the rigmarole.

I was giving Tom advice on how to improve his jumping technique on his scooter and this was quite a ridiculous situation, with my citrus appearance and a straining voice, like I was on stage as a failing drag act and everyone in the audience was just talking amongst themselves.

But Tom was taking my instruction extremely seriously and I was reminded of the times we used to go swimming in Forest Hill and how rotund and unlikely the very excellent swimming coach had seemed. It didn't appear to matter that I was wrapped up like oranges and lemons in my wheelchair, or my fractious castrato, because I had successfully managed to impart a small piece of information that had enabled him to achieve the scooter elevation he'd been looking for.

I suppose this was a little like those genre of movies best known through the *Rocky* franchise, in which the coach is some kind of misfit outcast who eventually comes good. Because this was once routine and normal, but now it's much more special than that. It's a *moment* of coming good and these are precious to me.

*

In his early life, Tom and I existed side by side, so that we made up our days together. In the mornings we'd look out at London, over bowls of porridge. In the foreground parakeets perched in the sycamores and someone's pigeons would swirl and circle over the nearby gardens. And from here, London spread out, as if the land were a vast map unfurled from the kitchen table. It was quiet at the top of our building, with only the clinking noises of breakfast and the frequent high-pitched sounds of a very young boy.

It amazes me to think I had this time with my son and that I had this opportunity. Just a dad and his young son, and I think I eased something in me by noticing and listening to him, so that just being aware of my interest felt like a different story in my life.

There's a lot of identifying that goes on for Tom. A lot of time spent layering knowledge and building up information. He figures out the world in this way – knowledge built upon knowledge – and I have travelled alongside him, navigating a social sea, observing children and play and patterns glistening in the spectral waters. Each day we were Darwin in the New World, taking out our notebooks, stepping out into the parks and the playgrounds – identifying and naming all the strange figures and shapes and permutations that moved in his life. If the three-year-old Tom saw a red spade attached to the end of an arm in a sandpit, we would work this out together, exploring the ways he might operate to become the person holding the red spade in this situation. Or if another child removed a green car from its appointed place in the design of his play, we'd examine the steps needed for the next time something essential was unexpectedly removed from his life.

But what now? What of the end of things? What of death, with our notebooks and our sense of wonder?

*

Tom must have been four when a starling flew into our loft through one of the tiny holes between the rafters. We heard its soft thudding, as it flew around up there – losing feathers, bruising itself, breaking little limbs. It had stopped by the time I had climbed through the hatch, and Tom was down below with his hands clutching the sides of the ladder and his mouth dropped open at the chin.

Back on the landing, I had the starling cupped inside my hand and the only movement came from the ruffling of chest feathers as they pushed against the fatty part of my index finger. I showed Tom briefly and then set off down the stairs, on my own, but by the time I reached the road the tiny pulsing in the starling's chest had stopped and it lay sideways on my hand. I didn't bury him. It was Thursday and the wheelie bin was full of rubbish, so I set his speckled feathers down upon a black and shiny plastic bin bag and closed the lid.

Tom was standing on the landing when I came back up and I told the story of what had happened, with something like the fanfare of the Wright brothers' maiden flight. I had moved through to the bathroom sink to wash my hands, and Tom had followed. As I scrubbed away with soap, I saw him as a reflection in the cabinet mirror, listening intently to my description of how this bird would now be flying overhead with his friends. I don't know what we did next but we dispersed. I think I closed the loft hatch and peeled some onions and maybe, through the kitchen window, stood and watched the parakeets. And then, a little while later, I heard another different sound. I went into Tom's room and there he was beneath the window, next to the cardboard space rocket we had made the week before, sobbing and sniffling into his lap.

*

In the early days, when it was just a limp, and even with Tom's neck craned up towards me, I knew enough, or had learnt enough, to say that my leg wouldn't be getting any better. And that's a hard thing to say to a pair of soft blue opioid eyes. Far easier to tap for a vein and say yes to biking together when the days get longer, or to swims off the river beaches that dot the mountainsides of central Portugal. To *not* say yes is a particular kind of arid route taken at a fork, one that offers perfect views of an alternative route descending into soft fluffy clouds or liquid pools the colour of translucent green sweetie wrappers.

I wonder how hard it is for a very young mind to comprehend that a body won't get better, and whether it is any harder or easier for an older mind. I don't think it registered with Tom when I then started responding that it wouldn't just *not get better* but that it would also get worse. We existed in the present tense, and even when I started having to use a walking stick – then graduated to a pair of crutches – for Tom I remained just exactly what I was: a dad who couldn't take him swimming over the summer because of a bad leg.

A month or two went by, and we had returned to the UK to live. I decided to give Tom the name for my condition and used my new expertise as an opportunity to explain the relationship between the brain and voluntary movement. I heard him trying the words out loud and, even though it came out as *mooto nuney disease*, the term sounded so much more serious and frightening than it ever had before. And I just wanted to take that language back. It felt like such a serious mistake to ever have imparted such language to someone so little, who I love this much.

However hard these experiences were with Tom, I was also able to draw on the medical expertise of the doctors from his imaginary island, and from those doctors working within its larger teaching hospitals on the smaller adjacent island. In the fifth year of Tom's life, Gill and I learnt a lot about these islands and came to understand that Tom and Jimmy's night-times were not spent asleep but on expediting their responsibilities as both mayoralty and chief engineers for these two island states. For quite some time, Tom was able to update me about the superior medical services on the islands and the advances that were curing limps in all their forms. Alongside this, engineers were constantly developing a wide range of off-road and flying wheelchairs that were making the experience of disability a lot more functional for people in my predicament.

But as time went on, and it became so clearly more than just a leg problem, and when I started moving so much less and doing so much less, I got the impression that innovation had declined on these islands – or that I was diseased to such an extent that even these highly skilled island engineers considered my condition beyond help. It's only possible to be a daddy with a bad leg for a limited amount of time. The present tense can only continue for a period of six months or so because, after this time, I realized I was existing within the *apart* tense, or in some kind of tense in which people or ideas languish until they are forgotten or disappear completely.

It's so easy to think that children don't know about death, even though they walk by spiders' webs all the time and see small things perishing. Things end all the time and yet people like me feel the need to lie to their children that a little bird isn't dying, when everyone knows otherwise. So many children see death around them every day, but I imagine they're capable of managing this information far more effectively than most adults, so that they can live alongside the knowledge of death whilst laughing at a fart or rolling a disused tyre down a hill for fun.

It was about two months ago, in our tiny cottage here, that Tom asked me if he was going to die one day. He had been crying in his bed and then came down to be with me, nestling himself on the blanket that was on my lap. And for that moment I'm grateful to that starling – and feel bad that I buried him in a wheelie bin – because I could see that my little son just needed to know that I was capable of being honest with him.

'What do you think?' I said.

'I think I will' was his reply.

'Yes, that's right,' I said. 'All of us die. It's part of life.'

Then I pulled the sides of the blanket in around him, and he quietly sobbed in this warm cocoon. And I thought of all the many children in the world, experiencing much harder lives than ours, who cannot be protected from this truth. And how the idea of death is part of Tom's life now. This boy I could feel in my arms, knowing inside that his father will die. The microscopic idea of it – expanding its cellular life – slowly becoming something that will be visible in his mind at exactly the point at which he needs it to be.

It was dark. It was raining outside, and in that moment the old stable beams creaked above us. It was just us and these tiny noises, and then it changed and we giggled off to bed.

How will the end of my life appear to my boy? In the long periods between connections I fantasize darkly about disappearing like granules of sugar in tea. Or that my absence might be registered like the absence of a treasured old cardboard go-kart – remembered fondly but no longer around. I'm frightened of the actual moment – when it's confirmed for Tom that I am dying, and that maybe it's easier to dissolve or to disappear on a Friday morning in a recycling truck. Because one day he will really know, and really say, and then loss will stretch out its lazy arms and legs and settle in.

*

I had trouble working out the number of birthday cards to stockpile for the boys. I wrote an article for the *Guardian Magazine* about writing thirty-three cards but my first draft contained various figures, so that at one point I confused my editor by also referring to the twenty-two cards, and later on that it would be twenty-eight. It had been an easy article to write, apart from the mathematics of it all, which was like one of those sticky strips that people hang up to catch flies but which instead attract tiny little floating anxieties.

The main difficulty was estimating the first of their birthdays for which I would be either dead or at the point when the act of passing a card to either of the boys might not be possible. These are quite profound sums and very different from those calculations involving apples and tenpence pieces through which I remember first learning arithmetic. Perhaps this is part of the point of learning maths, so that – at the end – you can easily use both hands to add up how long you have left.

There was a comments section attached to the article and I remember one subthread developed with readers trying to work out how I had arrived at the number thirty-three. I wouldn't have expected such curiosity but it's the idea of the future, or anticipating the future, and perhaps this is something naturally interesting or unsettling. In fact, I started the cards for Jimmy's fourth and Tom's eighth birthday, and with the way my body has atrophied since, I would say that this is exactly right and that I have yet again proved myself to be the world's foremost authority and expert on the subject of my own decline. My consultants are just the people left holding the clipboards.

My friend lost his father when very young and told me that birthdays were the worst of times. But quite a lot of time went by and I procrastinated about the grade of card required. It was only when I started to notice the tendons shortening on my right hand that I finally got under way, and when I first took a scalpel to the card, and set both my pens and paints out on the table, I could have been a lonely, peaceful figure, seated on a rock in a cave accessible only at low tides, located somewhere in the Pacific, perhaps a hundred miles from habitation. I had decided to use pages from a large watercolour pad, so the nap was grained and textured. When I held it between the fatty parts of my thumb and index finger it had more of a presence than I expected. And progressing with the cards felt like something very permanent, like the handover from one person to another, different form of presence.

I spent some part of my career working with young people in children's homes. And amongst the many hard circumstances I encountered, it seemed like the cruellest situation for a child to find themselves in a children's home whilst down the road their parents and siblings were living and sleeping in some normal terraced house like everybody else. And there were always different reasons for this surprisingly common situation but always the same clean circular hole through the centre of some young person's heart. And I can't imagine that hole ever heals over – that it remains in place with the air whistling through it with the sound of faraway family dinners. I suppose I mention it because mine will be a different kind of absence and a different kind of silence, but it's still absence and it's still silence. And because of this I wanted my cards to convey almost everything about love.

Jimmy liked all the pens and pencils and paintbrushes I had set out on the table. I looked down and saw his little arachnid fingers traversing the front lip of the desktop, so I rolled a colouring pencil towards his fingers and he padded off with it down the corridor. A few moments later he was back and giggling with joy at his light-fingeredness, prodding me in the bottom with the pencil to underline his victory.

The evidence of such unremarkable meetings is absorbed into walls and disappears from history. And that's OK for a boy who can remember and a daddy who isn't dying. But for Jimmy and me these innocuous moments happen and disappear, likes diamonds sliding down a crease of paper into a draining sink. That moment when I was weak and dropped my cutlery, and

Jimmy reached down and picked it up for me. Or those occasions when he decided I might want my hat and brought it to me, and when he sometimes tried to lift my trousers back up for me after I'd been on the toilet. This is it, before it dissipates through the walls. There is no after; this is no foundation. It doesn't continue on or roll forward like the torso of a snowman, compacting and gathering into fullness. After I was prodded in the bottom I realized I should record these moments, so that they didn't all disappear – that I should record this moment with the coloured pencil, and a different moment for each of Jimmy's cards. I also like the idea that this was exactly why I was being jabbed in the bottom – that my little son was peering up on to the table and telling me to stop with all the silly Daddy doodles, and all the love blah blah, and to get the evidence down instead.

Because if I were Jimmy, I'd want to know. What was it? What happened exactly, in that brief time? Was it real? Who was that man? Who was I?

I doodled less as the boys reached their late teens. I couldn't hold a pen or a brush by this stage, so the cards were typed and more like letters. From my desk I had a view of the pretty stone wall on the opposite side of the lane, a telegraph pole and the frosted tops of topiary from the large walled garden next door. I was writing to a broader Jimmy, with his looping bowl of a jawline; Tom was longer, with tufted wheat-coloured whiskers splaying out from the point of his chin. I had glimpsed these older boys before, when I was looking upwards from my watery world, seeing them moving around in the daylight up above ground. And I was existing ahead of them again now, walking around and touching the future bric-a-brac of their thoughts, having arrived in this quiet, unready future – like a street market in the hours before opening. I had made this time for myself to see what it could be and to reassure myself – wandering around and imagining, leaving little notes pinned to doors and attached to lamp posts, for my older sons to find in later years. And every one – every card I doodled and wrote and painted – was just a different-coloured way of saying that I would always be there, that I had tried in every way I could, and that I was sorry.

Fathers

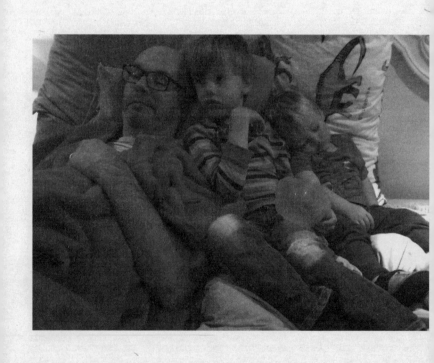

By the time my father reached old age his lifestyle had softened and it seemed that visiting him with my very young family was no longer the risk it once would have been. At this more genteel stage in his life he claimed to have grown weary of the more unstable female companions from his earlier years. His sexual interest had moved on and it was a subject about which he could become extremely animated. He never seemed to allow for the possibility that Gill might not be interested, or that a toddler might be staring up at him in that moment.

The walls of his home were decorated with large black-and-white framed prints of old ships and, interspersed between them, smaller framed prints of Victorian soft porn – women in petticoats with the corner of a buttock or breast just about revealed. When upstairs and seated in his favourite comfy chair, or with his apron on as he washed up, he'd find an opportunity to play a semi-famous reggae song from the 1970s in which a man expresses his infatuation for a woman with a larger than average sized bottom. He'd soon start singing along to the lyrics and waving his arms about, becoming particularly animated by those lines in which the object of the singer's infatuation is reassured by the singer that he is in no way intimidated by the size of her rear. Like many elderly people, my father lived alone and I suppose it was natural that he might store up his reflections or want to sing along to his favourite tunes. He'd become quite isolated in his dotage, with just one or two doting female visitors: his chiropodist and the woman described as 'cuddly' from the village clothes shop.

Sometimes he'd just prefer to sit back in his armchair and regale us with his most recent observations about the various large sized women he'd come across in the doctor's surgery or the hairdresser's. Occasionally he'd date a woman who conformed to this scale requirement of his, but mostly he just enjoyed chatting to them in shops or, best of all, finding one riding a horse, so that he could ever so slowly overtake her several times on a country road.

There were times when his eyes would glisten and he'd grow nostalgic for the 'wild women' of his 'bad old days'. He was sentimental about what he seemed to regard as this heyday of his romantic life, and was fond of recalling stories and women from this time. But when he did so, his adopted tone was one that might otherwise have been expected of an elderly widower recalling the sweetness of a courtship, from the 1940s perhaps, to a woman named Gladys.

*

If you don't know it, Spirograph is a children's toy made up of a pen and a set of plastic discs. It creates hundreds, or even thousands, of coloured concentric circles as a series of pretty patterns on paper. I mention this, not because I ever really had or used this toy, but because, if you were to track my father's route throughout our weekend visits, you would find Gill to be the centre-point of his perambulations – the place from which he would make repeated circular movements in to, and around, and back out again. If a coloured crayon had been attached to his feet, it would have made for a spectacular pattern.

Often he would appear before her offering a piece of memorabilia from his life, and sometimes he would arrive empty-handed with an anecdote: something recollected or perhaps drawing on the range of his social interactions with service providers and large female shop assistants. Occasionally he would ask Gill a question about her life, as if reading from cards compiled to assist a person's integration into polite society. I think he was delighted to find himself politely enquiring about the normal details of another person's life, even if he would seldom have time to delay the Spirograph long enough to take in the actual response to his enquiry. It always seemed like he found this part the least interesting feature of the exchange, and that he was also trying hard to perfect an air of casual nonchalance and the impression that his day was already overrun with tasks. At this stage in her life Gill hadn't yet handed back other people's overcoats and, given my slightly awkward and taciturn presence in this house, probably felt she had no choice but to accept the temporary draping of multiple parkas and mackintoshes around her shoulders. She would warmly welcome every approach, widening her eyes throughout the encounter and always asking the requisite number of follow-up questions. It was a simple arrangement and, watching the pattern, it looked a little like a woman throwing a stick for a dog as she tried to read her book. The pattern continued and he became so devoted that, within a few years, he declared Gill to be the daughter he always wished he'd had, and made the specific request that she refer to him as such.

If I make this sound in any way maladjusted, I really don't mean to. There probably isn't a person whose movements around their preoccupations wouldn't make a pretty enough Spirograph pattern, and which wouldn't grow more uniform and concentric with age. I was fairly stolid company during these visits and Gill, by contrast, quite delightful for a man who lived alone and had limited opportunities with people. She knew very little about the man he used to be and it never occurred to me to talk about any of that. I think he quite liked that Gill and I were *normal* people with *normal* lives and I'm glad that it made him feel good about himself. When we bought our flat he gave us a little money towards our deposit and, when we got married, he wore a nice suit to the wedding.

The first sign of trouble came when Tom was born. It's not that he didn't like the idea of having grand-children and, after visiting, he would request we follow up with photographic evidence of his interactions with Tom. From time to time he would remember actual details about Tom – his genuine characteristics and interests. And he cared enough to deposit money into a bank account for his grandson. But the main prob-lem with Tom was that he could not be relied upon to move out of the way of the Spirograph as it completed its round of patterns. It could be that the Spirograph returned to the centre and found a jigsaw or a nappy change under way. Or it could be that Gill or I were reading Mr Men books in the garden or that we'd taken Tom to the playground. These were awkward moments and what I remember is the magnified impression of his forbearance in the face of considerable disappointment; the sense that this was only one weekend in the year, and that it wasn't unreasonable to expect that it would be his alone, given that his grandson had the other fifty-one.

Occasionally he'd wince into the car alongside Tom and, if a trip were planned to somewhere that had interest for him, such as a steam railway or village fete, then everything would go off without trouble. But the idea of anything other than these destinations appeared to cause him real physical pain, so that he'd grimace or tug painfully at his ears – or he'd turn to face us at a 45-degree angle, making uncomfortable long low throaty noises. It wasn't just that he declined such opportunities, which would have been understandable, but something else took over in him that felt like an attempted bending of attention, away from his grandchild and back towards the established world of his own needs. If we were in the car, and we tried to settle on a destination or a parking spot, sometimes that would be so incredibly hard for him, and hard to dredge for a kind of coherent opposition. Just a frame lurching closer to the windscreen, his face screwed and contorting as he gripped the armrest or steering wheel, and a crooked forward-pointing finger urging us on to somewhere, anywhere.

*

I'm not sure if it's bad luck, or a familial quirk, but I realize I don't know one single old man who isn't some slanty-crowned despot in a comfy chair. It's a little sad for me that I don't know any old men who are different to this. I know they are out there. Or that some of them are out there. Because it looks hard to be old in this country. But when people trot out clichés about a *crisis in masculinity*, it's never old men who are mentioned. It makes me wonder if a little more infrastructure is needed or whether more children's playgrounds should be turned over in middle-class areas and made into something that could overtly celebrate and trumpet the lifelong achievements of this disenfranchised group.

Because I know so many men who have arrived at this point in their lives feeling frustrated and under-appreciated – and wondering why so much of the available attention is being commandeered by the very young. I see them carrying these brick-shaped feelings aloft, in high-up teetering gilded hods. And I don't think it necessarily makes them bad people, just that they seem to have haltingly arrived at this late place in their lives to find a vast gap has opened up for them, like a ravine, between what they had long ago expected and what was finally delivered.

They are often to be found, in gardens and living rooms, stamping and stomping in a kind of territorial dance – the very tall and the very small – fighting over who had this or that toy first. For example, in her retirement, my mum married for the first time and we stayed with her and her husband over the summer. Like my father, it's not at all that this man doesn't enjoy the company of Tom and Jimmy, or that he's not fond of them – because he quite clearly is – it's just that this regard is harder to maintain when children decide on their own particular forms of play, at their own appointed times. And so it proved when Jimmy – at eighteen months – failed to return a shoehorn that he'd been playing with. It wasn't larceny that we were initially aware of, and it only came to light when some of Tom and Jimmy's toys also started disappearing. It took some investigation to unlock the mystery but, one by one, the missing toys were found squirrelled away in various unfathomable locations.

My latest stepfather is nothing if not tidy, and this requirement – to have everything in its appointed place – was the initial tersely delivered rationale for hiding Tom and Jimmy's toys. I didn't find his response particularly measured, but I felt some sympathy for this elderly man, resisting the impact of his own debilitating ill health, and suddenly coping with the debris of children's lives. I hoped we could find a solution but, in that moment when the mystery of the toys had been revealed, it proved difficult to engage any kind of eye contact. Instead, the initially injured party stooped a few yards from us, working away with a duster for a prolonged period, at an area of the kitchen table about four inches square. He seemed perturbed by the surface and fixed his glare on its obstinacy. It was one of those unfortunate silences when a key party in a conversation remains temporarily distracted. But what happened next surprised us because, when he finally lifted his gaze from the table, the glare and perturbation remained, and even seemed directed in our direction. I think his right foot lifted ever so slightly and his knuckles pressed into the tabletop. When this downward force was released, his knuckles had whitened and his foot came back down with something like a stomp. He seemed particularly emotional and wanted to make clear that Jimmy had *started it* and that the provocateur in this situation had yet to return his missing shoehorn. I suppose we could have got the two injured parties together to sort this out, but it was 7 p.m. and Jimmy had already retired to his cot with a bottle.

*

Jimmy was just a few months old when we last visited my father and we were experiencing the familiar parental challenge of life with a second child. My father was also finding it challenging, but for slightly different reasons. Our lives were now stretched between the two young children, and the Spirograph was struggling to establish the clean consistent lines required for effective patterning. He would attempt his anecdotes exactly as he'd done before, but then a crying baby – or requests for more banana – would invariably result in a story left half finished. And I think he felt dismayed to see various mementos deposited amongst the wider debris of Lego and soiled nappies. I could see that he was becoming increasingly frustrated by the claims being made on Gill by his grandchildren. In the weeks leading up to our stay, Jimmy had been awake for long stretches during the night. Both of us had been lacking sleep and we were aware of not being great guests. We tried to explain, and the spaces at the end of Gill's apologies seemed tailor-made for some kind of sympathy but were instead filled with the dogged remains of half-completed anecdotes from earlier in the day.

The perfected air of nonchalance was the first to go, so that he became a little more strategic and observant. Within the first twenty-four hours the fluidity of the Spirograph gave way to a series of thwarted pounces.

He was becoming a much more peripheral figure and I could hear the dishwasher being emptied in a very noisy way. When the vacuum cleaner suddenly ploughed through the centre of a little family scene, it felt like a very specific point was being made.

The day before we were due to end our visit my father decided that he needed a large table moved. He hadn't previously brought up any furniture-moving requirements. The inspiration seemed to come from nowhere and was accompanied with a quite desperate sense of urgency. I could tell a lot was at stake, but Gill had fallen asleep with exhaustion and I was looking after both boys. I don't think he had factored in these environmental considerations because, by the time I could answer, he was already holding one end of the table with both hands.

'Do we need to do this now? You know that Gill's . . . ?'

I was holding Jimmy horizontally in the crook of both elbows, like an armful of firewood, and turned around, gesturing towards our bedroom with the top of his head. I don't know if it was the pain of an emerging tooth, but during these uncomfortable periods he required to be permanently held, very precisely, in a horizontal position, as if he was functioning as the replacement fluid bubble at the centre of a spirit level, and this was not at all about teething or colic, but instead about the process of putting up new shelving.

'Does it really need to be now?'

What is it about old men and tables? By this point he wasn't listening but was crouching low down, circling the edges of the table.

'I just can't put him down right now. Can it wait?'

I don't believe he answered, but I must admit to having been distracted by Tom's own frustration with a tricky stage in the construction of the fuselage of his Lego helicopter. Tom and I examined the instructions for a few moments and then I turned to Dad and wrestled Jimmy on to my hip.

'Look, I can take one end . . .'

I moved to grasp the table with my free hand, but I don't think the offer was sufficiently exclusive and my father abruptly swivelled a hundred and eighty degrees away from me. He goose-marched one leg forward, angrily flicking his chin and fingers upwards to the gods, as if directing the percussion section for his own private Wagner table-moving opera, and disappeared through to the kitchen.

A little time went by. With relief, I considered the table-moving safely suspended. By the time he had rejoined me in the living room, away from the table, I was giving Jimmy his bottle whilst watching Tom with his Lego. There was peace for a moment, and Gill was still sleeping. I looked around at the four of us. My father's gaze seemed fixed on some indeterminable spot, but the scene seemed almost the picture of a weekend away with the grandparents.

So it was a shock: the kinetic energy of this next moment was a shock. His arm thrashed at the air, snarling that something was for 'God's sake' – and then my very fit 83-year-old father leapt forty-five degrees up from his seated position. With his crimson V-neck camouflaged against the upholstery of his favourite soft chair, he momentarily resembled one of those highly adapted stick insects, invisible within their surroundings, that wait for days and then cantilever violently towards their prey.

This lithe old man lurched towards the table, grabbing one end of the beast as he vainly attempted some movement of its being towards his required location.

I looked over and remarked on this being the behaviour of a baby, but I think the words dribbled out and reached no further than the ends of my feet. Weak and old as he clearly was, having been frightened by this man at a very young age, it was always very hard not to feel overtaken by those ancient feelings.

And I don't think he was aware of my remark. He was sweaty and angry, and was particularly upset that a table leg had become snagged up in a ruffle of carpet.

'I only . . . I . . .'

He was panting and straining heavily at this stage, as if single-handedly attempting to manoeuvre a large reluctant mammal into some kind of pen.

At this point, Gill walked in and he snapped upright in his stance, flinging out an arm in my direction.

'He won't help me! He won't help me move the table!'

Gill looked at the table; she looked over at me.

'But he's feeding Jimmy!'

Looking back at this specific moment in time, I don't think it's possible to overestimate the momentary physical shrinkage his body underwent. His arm remained in position, aimed directly at me, and little thin pools of fluid floated across his eyeballs. He remained perfectly still, like someone in the immediate aftermath of being shot with a pistol in a stage play. Gill's simple and undeniably factual statement must have felt something like a bullet. And I think, in that moment, his full and unconditional love for his daughter-in-law hissed like a hot coal dropped into a bucket of water. She had observed him in this room and he must have wondered – must have looked down – just to check that he was wearing anything at all.

'I . . . I'm sorry . . . I . . . I need a . . .'

And with that he disappeared. To his office or his bedroom or somewhere.

It was about an hour later that he returned, and his response conveyed the brilliance with which he had configured his thoughts about our interaction into a simple, user-friendly concept. He resurfaced to make clear that, if we were to have any kind of meaningful relationship, from now on I must understand his need to be indulged. He'd worked out that I was missing this point. He came out to simplify matters and also to state, for the avoidance of doubt, that this requirement of his would never change.

Though for many years he had lived quite an unhealthy life, for the last decade or so he had lived as a vegetarian and was very trim and agile for his age. I mention this because, when he reappeared from his temporary isolation, he did not look in great shape. He was lurching, his shoulders curling forwards, his feet struggling to keep up with the sedentary pace of his upper body. The strain of the earlier events had resulted in a rapid physiological decline.

'You need to indulge me.'

This phrase continued. This simple phrase. So simple that it suggested an idea fully comprehended. Bruno Bettelheim, that great Viennese psychologist and thinker, once wrote about those moments in life when something is known to a person so completely that the words required to communicate this knowledge form with unusual clarity and precision. In this case, with my father, I think the obverse was true. He was wrestling a concept so obtuse that simplicity was all he was capable of.

'I'm not going to change. You need to indulge me.'

One of the problems of having been frightened by someone at a very young age is that anyone's anger in any situation takes you back to the original fear. And the corollary, certainly for me, was that my own anger had always been inaccessible, even in situations when that would be something quite natural and appropriate to feel. It's meant that I have long been regarded as calm and unflappable under pressure, when it's nothing more than adaptation – just carefully concealed fear dressed up as serenity.

So instead of dealing swiftly and decisively with my father's behaviour, I used the wrong kind of fire extinguisher. I tried to point out what seemed self-evident to me: that Gill and I have two very young children, that Gill had been up most of the night and that we were barely managing as parents. Unfortunately, this didn't work – as if I had used the foam extinguisher instead of the powder one, or water when I should have used foam – so that whatever had been combustible just became more inflamed.

There are those moments on a football pitch when a

player *loses it*. Maybe they feel unfairly treated by the referee – who has perhaps sent them off or awarded a penalty to the other side; maybe another player has done this or that to them and that other player has gone unpunished, and it all becomes too much for him. The oily cocktail mixing with his endorphins becomes something heady and spirited, and this foaming-mouthed, crimson-faced player leers beseechingly, this way and that, towards an invisible darkness where he feels his rage makes perfect sense; his arms flailing, fending off the unwelcome reasonableness of calmer teammates. Because throwing reasonableness at rage is like throwing water on to cooking fat. But why not? I throw reasonableness at a lot of situations. When I'm unreasonable, I throw reasonableness at that. When I should be unreasonable, I throw reasonableness at that too. So I took his arm; I appealed to his reason as he lurched from room to room, shaking me off. His arms flailed as I tried to get in front of him. I was just reasonable, which didn't get us anywhere. Eventually he sloped away and spent most of the rest of our stay either hiding in his bedroom with a cold flannel over his eyes, or playing his power-ballad mix-tape in the kitchen with the volume turned right up.

The next morning he finally stirred from his room as we started the car, and complained of a headache. Very reasonably, we showed him some sympathy. We very reasonably encouraged him to visit us (knowing that he wouldn't). We were very reasonable when thanking him for looking after us. He'd renovated the summer house for Tom to use during our stay and, very reasonably, we thanked him for this too.

And that would have been it. It could have ended there. Normally, it would have. All unhappy families work like that: someone says something they shouldn't, hits someone they shouldn't, fucks someone they shouldn't. Nothing much is said and then it happens again, and even less is said.

But in this case, I haven't seen my father again. I've spoken to him, and it's one of these conversations that effectively brought an end to our relationship – the one true, honest conversation I ever had with him. It was the point at which he ducked out of being a father. His heart was never really in it.

*

I've seen photos of my maternal grandfather and I look quite similar – the same long spine and hairless egg-shaped face. He separated from my grandmother when my mum was still a young girl and went to live somewhere in mainland Europe, from where he sent a letter saying that presents were on their way. But the presents never arrived and neither did he. She never heard from him again and no one mentioned him much after that.

In her old age, my mum has been keen to talk to me about her father and how celebrated he had been as a doctor. She will often talk about his notoriety and famous patients. Though he had been a non-practising Jew, she now considers this part of his cultural heritage and, therefore, hers too. She also tracked down descendants from the entirely new family he started several years after he'd left. And it always struck me that – in building this fuller portrait of her father – each and every new piece of acquired information affirmed something long neglected, as if all that really mattered was the accumulation, and not what may have been revealed about who her father really was.

There have been other cherished fragments of carefully restored information, cheerfully recalled – that he had a dog called Shit and that he boasted of his ability to 'break' women. And there are the treasured artefacts from his life: the book he wrote, that was 'ahead of its time', and his old cigar box.

And saddest of all, that he had always treated her as his favourite.

When I was seventeen, on New Year's Eve, three months after passing my driving test, I mowed down a motorcyclist on a country road. There were no street lights, and the motorbike had no headlights. The first I knew of our collision was a red windscreen and how it changed from one whole transparent piece to a vermilion mosaic. I stopped the car but the wing on the driver's side was concertinaed and I had to climb out of the passenger side. There was a crescent moon that night and I could only locate the motorcyclist from his series of low muffled sounds. Kneeling down beside him in the verge, I lifted his visor and was relieved to receive a breathy request for his asthma inhaler. But as I went to search his pocket I noticed that his arm had come away at the elbow. Then I noticed he had only one leg and that his foot was missing from the other. The police arrived shortly after. And about thirty minutes later, in the back of a police car, a kind policeman told me that he had died.

I often think of this man in the verge. I think of how he talked to me, oblivious to the catastrophic damage that had been done to him, believing that all he needed was the inhaler in his pocket. And I also think of my mum, as she lies grinning in a verge after the carnage of this one-time father – the grass growing up in long tufted clumps around her – still believing that what she needed was the idea of his eminency, and his old cigar box.

*

Four months after that visit to my father's, I needed to phone from Portugal to tell him my news. For some reason, I worried this might be hard for him, so I'd arranged for someone to be there when I phoned. But over the course of the conversation I got the impression that something else was on his mind, or perhaps that he was having to accommodate something sticky lodged in-between his gums. His reaction to my news sounded strangely formal, like sentiments a visiting dignitary might express.

I don't think this makes him a heartless person. I know that he's as much a feeling person as any other. Three years before, his dog had died and I think this loss had remained so profound that it was hard to feel the loss of a son. Some years before this, there had been an occasion when he astonished me by bringing out a huge bulging photo album. Gill and I sat beside him as he opened its creaking leather cover. I could see that it was a record of much of his life, and there were photos of me I never knew existed, but, with the manner of his flick-through, there was very little time to dwell on anything – as if he were looking for something very specific in a catalogue. Eventually, a double spread remained open and his fingers reached in, tenderly feeling the glossy image of a dog he once owned. Several pages further on, and there was another one. He looked at both of us, in turn, his eyes watering over as he recalled the names of various Border collies, along with touchingly detailed descriptions of their different qualities and features. Eventually, either it all became too much or he ran out of dogs (it wasn't clear which). The album snapped shut and was returned to a cabinet drawer.

I could hear him at the other end of the line, searching along his bookshelves for an emotional response to my diagnosis. He probably knew something was called for but couldn't quite locate the motivation for it, and the conversation soon petered out, with a kind of strange, sad flatness, as if there hadn't really been any need for it in the first place. I wasn't fully aware of this at the time but, from comments he later made, I realized how painful it was for him that I was taking currency away from his own minor ailments, and I suppose that *would* make someone feel a little less sympathetic. He could see his own death being upstaged somewhere on the horizon, which wasn't at all what he wanted.

I know that when I describe my father, it might be hard to understand why I would have persisted with the relationship. I now realize I should have pulled away many years, or even decades, before. But at the time I believed he would come good and I think, had he been a younger man, or less isolated in the way he lived, he may well have done. When I was seventeen, and had my terrible car accident, I remember him wrapping his arms around me and, in that moment, I felt comforted. In that moment, he had been my father. It had taken a collision; sometimes it does. But I knew it was possible. Something in me still believed that. And also that I needed it; or that I needed him.

I thought of what he would have done for one of his dogs if they had fallen ill – that he would have stayed up all night by its side, holding a beaker of water to its mouth; that he would have taken his jacket off and tucked it gently in around his beloved companion. His life was full of such kindness and care towards animals. This was really who he was. I choose to believe this. And I feel sad that I never really knew this different man but sadder still for him, for what was squandered in his life.

In the weeks that followed, we prepared to come home for Christmas, and my father was keen to visit. It felt like something positive from him and, when we discussed this meet-up, I naturally inflated the extent to which we were all looking forward to seeing him. I thought this would offer the most helpful platform for our conversation.

'What happened, Dad, when we came to see you . . .'

I paused, considering how direct I felt able to be.

'Yes?'

'That can't happen again.'

'What do you mean?'

'I should have said at the time . . . how upsetting that was.'

'Yes, I know.'

'Do you?'

'Thirty seconds, it would have taken.'

'What would?'

'I only wanted it moved a few feet.'

I did feel deeply sorry for him. There was something very weak and very old in his voice. I probably knew him and understood him quite well in this moment, and maybe that's a kind of closeness, even if he is unlikely to have felt this way. But in recalling what was then said, I should add that this conversation with my father took place amidst the calm aftermath of those watery days following my diagnosis. And Tiago the Engineer, with his vast hydroelectric power plant, and the water that kept coming. I was listening to this man on the phone, with his lingering feelings of hurt and injustice, and it felt like this – or *thought* felt like this: that this moment of realization was like hundreds of tiny silver ball-bearings, which had long been jostling and circling endlessly inside me – for years maybe – around the deep sides of a large funnel, and had suddenly changed momentum and curved their gravitational direction downwards, rolling downwards in unison, out through the spout, with a rumble and a swoosh and a zip.

'You mean you're still upset about the table?'

'I don't know why you were being so difficult about it.'

In some ways, it's surprising that my father listened to everything I then had to say, but I think all bullies hate themselves and all they really want is for someone to stop them. And I don't think I did that but, for the briefest of moments, I think he wanted to listen.

What followed was something of a role reversal because I spent several minutes talking about matters that were so clearly of no interest to him. I explained what it felt like to *want* to live in a way that makes your children feel safe and cared for. I said I felt sorry for him (never helpful in a conversation) that he never had the opportunity to feel this way about his life. Sometimes people like a bit of sympathy and sometimes they don't. In this case, I wasn't sure because he didn't say anything. But then I realized that I hadn't actually *asked* a question, and that he may have considered what I had to say as a complete statement that didn't warrant an answer.

So I decided to ask him, quite unsuccessfully, what he thought life might be like for Gill and Tom and Jimmy over the next few years. But I think what happened is that he'd become overused to my statements, and missed my slight change of inflection; either that, or he was employing some kind of unwritten rule limiting the time allotted for one participant to be allowed to select the subject matter of a conversation. I imagine this would be like one of those time counters used in serious chess contests but, in my father's case, it would be a piece of hardware only issued to his opponent. Because, instead of replying, this was the point at which he alerted me to the presence of his bucket list, which he appeared to feel was being overshadowed by my terminal condition. He expressed some concern about this, and reminded me of his age. Eighty-three. And only a few years left, apparently. I hadn't known about his bucket list. I wonder what's on it? Because it seemed that a little too much time had been spent on other people's misfortune and I think he needed to express how short-changed he was feeling in not having had the opportunity to tick off any of his items.

It's interesting that conversations are such highly efficient structures. I suppose we are social animals and everything we say to each other has a kind of melodic logic. It may have seemed that my father had changed the subject but, in bringing up his bucket list, he was very astutely addressing the other question I had wanted to ask, which was whether he still felt that I should be indulging him. The notion that I should be had nibbled away at me since our visit but, since my diagnosis, it had become a much more pressing question. I was fairly sure that his concern for his bucket list had indirectly answered my query, but I decided to ask the question anyway, in a purely rhetorical sense. And what surprised me was the controlled anger that came out when posing this question to him. It wasn't something I'd ever presented before, certainly not on any occasion when it had been warranted. It felt a bit like I was spitting the question out – expelling perfectly proportioned pockets of lung capacity through the tiny gap between my bottom and upper teeth. And his response to this question – rhetorical or otherwise – was an uncharacteristically lengthy silence.

So much of what we say is self-evident. A lot of what is said never really needs saying. And this was definitely the case when I then reassured my father that I wasn't frightened of him any more. He claimed not to know that I ever had been (which he probably didn't) but remarked that he considered it an incredibly rude thing for me to say. This struck me as quite an odd response; the kind of response that causes the recipient to look upwards at a 45-degree angle, as if pondering a taxing piece of mental arithmetic.

But of all the things I said to him in this conversation, I think the statement that riled my father most was telling him that I loved him. Actually, I was unfairly provocative because I repeated this a couple more times. And when he emailed me following the conversation, it was these repeated statements that proved most controversial. He couldn't seem to square these statements with what had preceded them. And that's a shame, because I couldn't have made them without the details that had preceded them.

I don't know what I expected, but this proved to be an ending. The passing of time hasn't helped. Something had been *done* to him. I think that's how he feels, and always has, it seems to me. But I suppose the last thing I would say about my father is how resourceful he has always been, amidst the carnage of other people's lives. I find that quite impressive, in a way. And whilst I feel sad for what he has denied himself, I worry less because of this. I picture him at home, having redrawn the circle of his life, and living passably within it. With his memorabilia, and his soft-rock mix-tapes; the visits from his chiropodist and the 'lady friend' from the local clothes shop.

And maybe with a little caterpillar he has stopped to notice, as it slowly makes its way across his garden path towards the fresh green leaf – lying exactly at the mid-point of this journey – that a kind and gentle elderly man has laid down for its refreshment.

When I reflect on the way my father's life has ended up – absenting himself, as he largely has, even from contact with Gill or his grandchildren – I wonder if this is really what he wanted all along. Not the intrusion of people making claims upon his life, but these little things instead. And also that he has succeeded in that rarest of achievements, in finding for himself a kind of peace.

What Dying Really
Feels Like

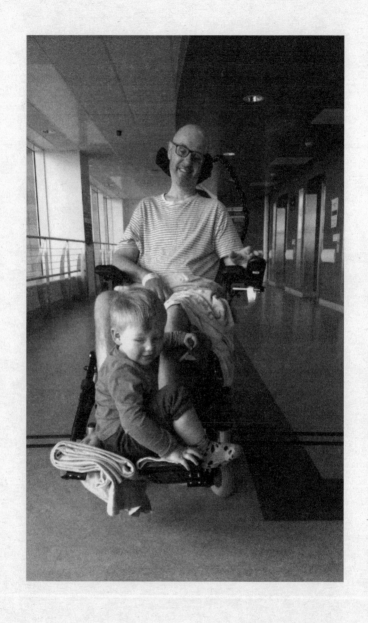

I'd been wheeled back through the ward on a commode with my naked bottom hanging out through a hole. And from behind my curtain the nurses then hoisted me to standing, with my pants and trousers around my ankles. I now have limited rotation in my trunk and shoulders, so I'm fully reliant on others for help. One of the nurses was kneeling down behind me with a bowl of hot soapy water, and the other nurse – the one in control of the hoist – had dropped her hip, and was waiting there as she leaned lazily with her hand on the bony rim of her pelvic girdle, like it was the lip of a garden fence and she was taking a break from gardening. A brace was protecting my neck weakness and I was able to look out through the long window behind her, at the view of Headington Cemetery and the scuffed flat greenery of Elsfield beyond.

This had been my second experience of having my bottom wiped, but now I'm well into double figures.

I went from the hospital to the hospice, where it's not unknown for four nursing staff to be present as I'm wheeled to my en suite in the standing hoist. Already at a height of six foot three, the hoist platform elevates me a few inches higher than normal and it all feels quite conspicuous. I'm attached to the hoist by a belt and, with my neck collar, I can feel a little of what the manacled King Kong must have felt, transported by ship initially, and then paraded on the back of a lorry through the streets of New York.

Once I'm stood over the toilet, someone drops my pants to signal the beginning of one of the more technically challenging procedures here: to locate me on the toilet seat in the same way that skilled parachutists try to land in a circle. If I were in their position, it's a procedure, and an act of teamwork, I would relish – and a lot of it is completed with subtle nods and glances, as is the case for a lot of team sports. It's a two-person operation, this one, with the first participant taking up a crouched position, with my hips in both hands, to guide me on to the white oval target. But this is not the skilfulness that should be trumpeted here, in the same way a person who simply *dunks* a basket after receiving a high long-distance pass should really be the least celebrated player in this particular basketball move. The nurse at the helm is the *player*, because they have to wheel the hulking hoist apparatus with one hand, whilst operating the down button that actually lowers my bottom precisely into place. If another couple of nurses are present, they tend to be little more than spectators lingering in the doorway.

One of the added levels of difficulty is that the toilet in my room appears to have been custom-made for a tiny old lady, so that when I land in place my small termite mound is only visible momentarily before sinking into the soft pillow of my scrotum. There's no real way to preserve dignity in the situation and I have completely given up on that. To begin with, most of them had been aware that I had that requirement for some kind of dignity, and had taken the opportunity – once they'd lowered me onto the seat – to cover me up, but after a while it had all felt a bit futile, and now none of us bothers with any kind of pretence. Given that my naked bottom is lowered so sportily into place on such a regular basis, it doesn't really matter what happens at the bottom.

I'll usually remain here for several hours – strapped in place, my neck braced – with hot drinks passed to me at intervals, and a little workstation established to my left-hand side. Yesterday I spent six hours of my fiftieth birthday sat on this hospice toilet, with a bottle of good Scotch wedged between my knees. As my body declines, the intestinal tract also loses impetus, and its contents slow to a crawl, like the stinking, stagnant waters of an urban industrial waterway. I can't really tell what deficit is killing me with this disease – it's probably respiratory failure – but if I think about daily discomfort, or even fear, the great peril is further down, where my colon has become the repository for fallen masonry, discarded shopping trolleys and an unwanted leather sofa.

*

I was in hospital to have a piece of plastic tubing threaded through my gut, and out through the wall of my abdomen. From this new orifice, the tubing runs for about eight inches and I tape it to the side of my belly to stop it dangling. A little tap fits on the end, so that the transparent tubing offers a window into the gemstone colours of gastric juices: a flowing syrupy nectar cordial flecked with flaming orange deposits. It's like some fancy inside-out architectural marvel, neatly combining interior and exterior features. Or maybe an extension of the popular taste for exposed features: exposed beams, exposed brickwork and now exposed gastric juices.

Initially I wondered if the tube had been a mistake. I was able to keep it taped up, as if it was a piece of body art, whilst continuing to consume vast amounts of stinky soft cheeses. There has been something sad and end-of-season about my recent period of make-believe gluttony, fooling myself with selective fine dining, even if I am staying in a hospice – as if I am a person without any swallowing difficulty at all, and I'm something quite the opposite: a gourmand or, even better, a *bon vivant*.

But the real experience is so stressful, or even a little scary, for anything that isn't soft and squishy. I've become aware of how slick and smooth the swallowing process usually is because, in feeling this loss of functioning, I am now more aware of the effort it takes for any tiny morsel to make its way towards digestion. The whole experience is so sluggish, and makes me think of disaster movies from the 1980s, in which a frightened group of survivors face a labyrinthine route to safety, through a disastrous inferno or the capsized hull of a luxury cruise ship. This might sound melodramatic, but my trachea has become something like a dreadful dark precipice for peas or fragments of pastry or grains of rice. The wrong material regularly makes its way down my windpipe and I'm told, given my declining lung capacity, that the infection risk from this misdirection represents my most likely cause of death from this disease. I can feel it precisely when something in my gullet is at risk: a morsel languishing in the wrong place, at the opening of my trachea. At this point I slow my breathing right down, concentrating on subduing my inhalations until this fragment makes its way on to a place of safety. It's the point in one of these films when the party of survivors traverse some terrible drop and the hero of the movie hangs back to take each one by the hand, encouraging them not to look down, until someone does.

I was told, once I started using my tube for my nutrition, that it would gradually start to change colour: to something surprising, like black or pink; something opaque, masking all the juicy backwash. Apparently there's no predicting the colour but, if I could request it, I would opt for the colour of both gangrene and grass.

About a week ago, very shortly after having the tube fitted, this possibility was brought forward, quite suddenly. It was the moment in this disaster movie when the narrow gap above the ravine opens up, and almost nothing can make its way through, or when a huge risky leap is required. I had expected this to happen more gradually, not huge slabs of the precipice crumbling away at my feet. But with further gradations of change now almost impossible, actual food is quickly becoming even harder for me. I can still sip soup through a metal straw or, with a teaspoon, still eat the gooey cheese that friends keep dropping in here as a gift, but anything more than this now feels like an act of recklessness. I do wake with forgetfulness, or drift into impulses for this or that favourite food, but instead of this I've now experienced my first moment of looking down at boring creams and whites and beiges piping through into my belly. These are no longer the colours of danger, but I can see that my transparent tube shows subtle signs of misty discoloration, and all the excitement and all the expectation is now to find out what colour I will become.

*

A few days ago I heard what I thought was a young girl sobbing in the corridor outside my room. I'm in what the nurses refer to as the green corridor, just opposite the chaplain's office. I don't see any of the other patients because most are too unwell to leave their rooms, but I see the families and, when I heard the crying, took a few moments to make certain that this voice couldn't belong to a patient. The crying went on for some time and I became worried the girl was on her own.

I have to be hoisted out of bed now, so it would have been completely impossible for me to help. I pressed my buzzer for one of the nurses to come and it took several attempts to explain that I didn't need help myself, but that I was worried about the girl outside. Then I heard the story – that this was a seven-year-old girl whose father was very ill in the room next door. Her mother was with her, and she was being looked after, or so I was told. The girl had come out into the corridor, where there is a table and chairs and a large brown teddy bear. Having imparted this information, the nurse then left with all her usual and admirable cheerfulness, as if I had instead rung to ask the name of a capital city for a quiz, and that she had been able to supply me with this detail. I think there's too much death in this place and not enough death everywhere else. Death is too common-place here for grief to fully open its wings. There's too much equipment, too many walls, too many trolleys carrying cake and pills and mashed potato. A little girl sobs in the corridor for her father, and it's just a function of what happens here.

A few minutes later and I heard the sobbing again. Whoever this girl was, she didn't seem entirely happy with what was coming out; or perhaps she was worried that the terrible violence of her tears might be considered naughty and was trying to catch them in both hands and stuff them back inside. The anatomy of crying is so much clearer in audio alone and these tears sounded like they were connected to a new chrome pump that was powerful but squeaking with its newness. It was clearly the first time this particular pump had been properly put to use.

And the worry surfaced – or a kind of panic, which had been there from the start – that this wasn't a seven-year-old girl; that it was Tom; that it had been Tom all along, crying outside my door.

I came here after the feeding tube was inserted because I'm now too immobile for our temporary home. I'm waiting for work to finish at the bungalow, and I'll be back with Gill and Tom and Jimmy. There's a little strip of glass on my bedroom door that people push their noses to: nurses and doctors and cooks and the volunteers who bring the tea. And I'm 'ducky' and 'luv' and 'honey' and even 'sweetheart'. My pillows are turned, my wee bottle emptied, my feeding tube flushed through with water. This is it. This is all of it. And learning new skills, like how to pee upwards or that it's actually possible to drink hot tea through a straw. It makes me wonder if what I'm experiencing isn't dying at all, but some kind of procedure.

In some other cultures it's not uncommon for paid mourners to be present at a funeral, or for the guest list to be stretched so that distant connections with an overt talent for grief can be encouraged to attend. That's what's missing; that's who should be present here: those capable of flapping their long dangly sleeves and gnashing their teeth; wailing and beating their chests, as they stick a thermometer under an armpit or fold the hospital corners on a bed.

And then it would be possible, or normal even

– something embraced and understood – to be a seven-year-old girl in a corridor, really crying for the loss of her father.

*

There's a moment when putting any bunch of flowers in a vase and one of the stems breaks, and it's propped up in the bunch as if nothing much is wrong. My neck started weakening a couple of months ago and only from this experience I've realized how central it has been to a lot of my life. It's not something I would ever have considered but I can see, from being a *pain in the neck* or just having a *millstone* around it, that the central importance of necks is widely understood. Otherwise, I wouldn't be able to *risk my neck*, or *stick my neck out* even further, before *catching it in the neck* for having such a *brass neck*.

There is something floppy, like a rag doll, in the way my neck supports my head. And the way I move and hold myself is dependent on angles, otherwise my head flops forwards or backwards or side to side, and someone has to lift it back up, like they are on the beach, balancing two pebbles on top of each other.

As she tried to lift my legs on to the bed, one of the nurses referred to me as dead weight. I think it just slipped out, as she struggled with my two calves, one in each hand. My body mass is now far more attuned to gravitational forces than it ever has been; far more so than for most people. I'm not cheating gravity with all my little movements, because even waving goodbye to someone, or pointing towards a beautiful flower or plant in the garden, is just another way of cheating the natural laws governing how solid objects are drawn to each other, and away from, in any given space. My pure existence in space precludes me from even the quite simple and everyday cheat of sitting at the table to have dinner, because sooner or later my torso and neck will express their gravitational obedience and my forehead will drift ever downwards towards my plate of soft foods, or to the centre of the earth, whichever should be closer.

I have often had a child's thought with broken stems: that maybe I could tape them up and they would be OK. A strip of Sellotape around the bruised blue line of the stem. Because it can seem like the shape is still there, and that it would otherwise be wasteful. But something fundamental has been lost, something connected and fluid about this structure that can't be fixed.

*

When I started writing this book my right hand was already weak, and I wondered if I might finish by typing with only one hand, or that I might need to dictate the final chapters. But, by a strange and counter-intuitive quirk, the act of typing has actually become easier over the last couple of months. The ligaments on my right index and middle fingers are shortening, causing them to curl around like two stubby question marks. They hover in this shape over the keyboard, so that when I type they resemble two birds pecking at seed, making the act of pressing keys that bit more efficient than it has been for quite some time.

I've experienced three genuine periods as a writer. The first was when I was nine years old and serialized the great Egg and Bacon wars. The eggs and their allies – the fried bread and sausages – fought a series of bloody battles against an alliance of fried tomatoes, mushrooms and bacon; and each of the key battles were set down by me over a period of months. I even found an audience in those early days, as I stood at the front of my class and read from my chronicles over a number of Friday afternoons.

The next period was in my early thirties, after I finished university as a mature student. I was trying to write screenplays, but this only became creative when I started writing for theatre. I had no significant professional success, but I experienced creating something that felt true and complete. These were the early years of my relationship with Gill, and the comic exploration of writing these plays felt like another way of understanding myself. The best of them – *Skinny Man* – was about a forty-year-old man who has gone to live on the rocky promontory of a deserted Hebridean island. In the three acts of the play he is visited, in turn, by the three different women in his life – his mother, his ex-fiancée and his sister – who each try to convince him to return, whilst breaking down the grandiose ideas he has cultivated about himself. He has mistaken his flaws for some kind of greater purpose, and I suppose the play is about the different ways that men fail to understand women.

The achievement of writing lifted my energy and confidence. I enjoyed being myself, which I never had before, but once the plays had been written I became too dependent on other people's opinion of my work to live happily with what I was doing. *Skinny Man* got me an agent, and got near to production on various occasions, but was never produced. In the face of that elongated setback, I wasn't as resilient and resourceful with my career as I needed to be, and I eventually lost confidence. I became happier when I stopped writing plays and left that life behind. So many years went by, in which being a dad became the important and creative focus in my life. It proved to be a better life for me, but I knew I was waiting to write again; I just didn't know what or how or who for. Then I was diagnosed, and everything was resolved.

I never knew who I was writing plays for: audiences, literary managers, artistic directors. I made it into an impossible task and frustrated myself into depression. But when I set out writing this book, it was for Tom and Jimmy, and I understood what was needed. Now that my respiratory function is failing, I realize I'm unlikely to be alive when this book is published and, however scary this is, it connects me to the original purpose of writing it. I'm unlikely to know anything about the public life of my story; only that I have written a book that will sit on a shelf for many years until my two sons are old enough to read it. This is where the book started and there is something reassuring in knowing I am returning to this.

*

The lights on the ventilator I now use at night remind me of a car dashboard. The function buttons display in bright white; the interface in fluorescent royal blue. The flow of oxygen vibrates the concertinaed plastic tubing, swooshing through the night. And the rubber housing fits snugly inside my nostrils, so that my nose, in isolation, benefits from what feels like a constant nighttime supply of A/C.

Lungs *feel* essential. They're right there in the midst of things. Other more complex organs exist, but I don't imagine their functional decline can be felt and noticed in the same intimate way. I'm aware that my inhalations stop at a certain point, and that my chest cavity doesn't push up and out as it used to do. If this were a new Hoover, I would replace the bag; or if Tom and I were pumping up his bicycle tyre, I would assume we hadn't properly connected the pump to the valve.

It's happened quite quickly with my lungs or, more specifically, with the muscles around my lungs. And it's surprised me because I expected this deterioration to be a few months away, and that when we arrive in our new home I would continue to be someone observing points along a route: the shrinkage in my willy, my new disability equipment, the changes in my relationships. But some of this more serious decline has happened unexpectedly, as if I had fallen asleep en route and been woken by an unfamiliar platform announcement.

I suppose I'm recording something different now. It's the first time that medical professionals have begun initiating conversations about *value* and dignity in dying. It feels like I am in the midst of preparation for something. Various documents have been handed to me and various choices presented – a bit like the baggage and car-hire emails received in the days before flying.

But one of the problems I have is that Jimmy has made my mobile hoisting device into a portable ice-cream factory. This started at the farm cottage and has continued here, with his visits to the hospice. He keeps offering me different flavours and the supply is inexhaustible. It's just very hard to make decisions that might limit my life expectancy when there is such a plentiful supply of imagined ice cream, in virtually any flavour I want. It's simply impossible to think about dignity in death with Jimmy being wheeled in, swirling and slurping with a double butterscotch scoop in a chocolate-dipped waffle cone, which I can eat without any difficulty right through the plastic casing of my oxygen mask.

*

I find death so interesting that I wish I had known about it earlier. I've been to funerals before, but I don't think I ever picked up that this would also happen to me one day. But now I realize how essential this information is and that any journey, no matter how enjoyable, loses value without a very clear sense that it will, at some point, come to an end.

There are so many clues that life doesn't go on for ever, but I know from my own experience that it's possible to keep dead bodies in boxes of different kinds, so that they remain out of conscious view. For this reason, I can see that my diseased body presents a difficulty for many of my visitors. I can see it in their faces as they first see me, as if Gill hasn't just handed them a cup of tea, but a grenade instead. They are like little birds hopping in front of me. Or they suddenly find their shoelaces need adjusting, or that the handle on their mug needs rotating twenty degrees or so. Just these little distractions, so that I can be made into anything other than a person before them who is simply dying. I think the conversations they are having are not with me but with themselves; conversations in which they reassure themselves that they are not the ones now dying. Or that death is not a thing at all; that I am somehow different in this way.

It's frequently the case that a tall pedestal appears between us and I'm expected to climb up on to it so that I can be elevated to a safe distance away. It's not always clear why, or even if there is any reason, and I don't tend to see much of these people. They're usually in and out of the door in very little time, chucking my pedestal into the boot of their car and accelerating away quite quickly. I get messages occasionally, to say that I continue to be a profound inspiration in their lives and that I must keep fighting.

Despite the severity of my disability, and that Gill remains my sole carer – whilst also caring for two very young children – it's common for visitors to respond to our difficult circumstances by squeezing or stuffing as many of their own needs as they can into any available space. This has been most noticeable with family – as if they feel the need to make up for my future absence by pre-loading opportunities for their own capital achievements to be recognized. In this way, grief feels less like the impending loss of a beloved, and more like an outbreak of looting. It must have been exactly this kind of phenomenon that took hold of one relative, with his surprise offer to show us his new sports car. Perhaps this felt like a particularly helpful offer, and that he had found a perfect opportunity to make a difference with his new toy.

I know there isn't any malign intent in all this need – just that whole bootloads of it exist in people, who then assume, because we are in a crisis, that our home accepts this particular kind of fly-tipping. Because the thought that death might actually be possible in a life seems to create waves of panic, causing certain people to stretch their arms around possessions, in search of something permanent and solid – made of chrome, perhaps, or moulded polypropylene, or teak. I see so much of this now that I am dying: that my fragile body is glimpsed and the onlooker's two eyes spin around like a slot machine, coming to rest with two portraits of their own image and the promise of a payout that never comes.

One of the startling experiences has been noticing

how hard it is for my mum to care for me, or her inability to loosen and show some tenderness; how unnatural this now feels for her; how she reaches in to care for me or Gill – her grandchildren too – but always misses with her grasp and finds herself instead. I dread her presence, for the horror that ripples across her face whenever she sees me. She sees the care and love that's shown to us by others, but a little voice inside sees jars of different-coloured sweets on high-up shelves; something little and sugary that she's needed all her life but never received. There's an envy in her care that I know she doesn't want but can't prevent. And it's clear to me – now that I am weak and vulnerable – that many people have spent so little time being cared for themselves that it has now become impossible for them to really care for anyone else.

I see that we have all been part of something social and familial that just doesn't work, and that it doesn't work at the exact point in time when it should work best. Of the two most recent deaths in my family, the first wasn't even marked with a funeral and, with the second, potential mourners were encouraged not to take time out of their busy lives – that it wasn't expected or necessary or, it seemed, wanted. Whenever I *have* been to funerals in this country, they have taken place in some tiny crematorium chapel, with five or six sallow-faced mourners crammed into something that resembles a swimming-pool changing cubicle. And then everyone spills out into the local drive-through, so that what passes for collective remembrance is some grey liquid sloshing in a cup stand somewhere on the M25. To conduct relationships in this way is like enjoying books but always missing out the last five pages – so that births and marriages are celebrated, but death is acknowledged with, at best, an email.

I can make most sense of this thought by reflecting on the widow of my Canadian uncle, whose warmth and tenderness has been in such striking contrast. It hasn't been necessary to actually *be* with this distant elderly relative, only to be in correspondence, but still to feel that her arms are all around us – caring and climbing into the different experiences that Gill and our children are living through. And when I think about why she should be acting so differently in our lives, I can see that she already knows about loss – how she loved my uncle for many decades, and has been living with his loss for almost two decades more. I don't imagine that loss frightens her, or feels irrelevant to her, because it must have become something so familiar and known and lived with.

A striking number of the friends who remain close to us are from Irish families – from a culture in which the experience of loss and grief is more closely woven into the social fabric of communities. Within such a culture perhaps it's not necessary to be an elderly widow, living daily with giant loss, because the stories of loss have become more widely shared and accepted. And it therefore becomes more natural to be a person reaching out to someone at the end of life. So I wonder if this is how families or communities or whole societies fail – that what is lacking, or what seeps away, is the necessary vastness of both love and loss. The beautiful volcanic, glacial, tidal landscapes that might otherwise remain visible in the far distance of life are just ignored, or construed as fiction, or tidied away in a drawer for later. These awesome lands are inevitably arrived at, of course, but never appreciated for their majesty, just fallen into, or over the edge of, in the midst of a holiday or a television programme or a tasty snack.

People have divided in life like oil and water, between those who arrive at our door with flimsy boxes full of their own packaged-up needs, and those more fortunate individuals who feel a comfort or familiarity with the idea of loss, and who must have felt, at some time in their lives, that their vulnerabilities have been taken care of. Certain lives seem less bound by fear, and it's remarkable to notice this difference between people: how some come into our lives and seem to notice so much more; people who visit us and take the time to imagine and observe, or who notice that the dishwasher needs emptying, or those who just kneel on the rug and spend their time with the boys so that Gill can sleep or take a shower.

I'm grateful to these friends who sit with me and hold my fragile hand without recoiling. I'm not sure that I would ever have been one of them – that I ever had the understanding or confidence to be this stature of person. If it's possible to be inspired at the end of life, as well as at the beginning, then that's what has happened to me. I've glimpsed other people's purpose in how to live and die, and now this is part of the story for my own little family. They are cosmologists, in a way, these people, for measuring the time it takes for light to flood from distant stars; which is just another way of knowing that any life is short. And that, measured from this distance, my own life isn't any shorter than their own.

*

I was planning to have my ashes scattered in Sydenham Hill Wood – the place I most associate with Tom and with my experience of being a father. On the edge of the wood is St Stephen's Church, where Gill and I were married. But then someone told me I could be buried in the wood, very close to us here, in Hampshire.

I was driven down to the site on a wet December afternoon by a man who used to design luxury hand-bags in the East End. He was reintroducing native trees and plants to the wood, and natural woodland manage-ment, which is something I don't know about but which sounds like a good thing. It was raining heavily when Gill and our guide got out to look. I watched Gill cross around in front of the car and disappear out of view to my right. I can't turn my neck, but they would have disappeared in through a clearing in the wood to look at the site. I sat looking out through the rain at the field below, and a few minutes later heard a car door open behind me and next to me, and two wet figures climb-ing in.

When Gill and I first wrote our wills, we requested that our ashes be scattered in the Indian Himalayas, which is not a decision that anyone with a balanced idea of their own mortality would make. It sounds like an option you might select for a wager or for something that has an outside chance of occurring. It was Gill who initially liked the idea of a woodland grave close to where we live. Bluebells grow on the site and I am planning to have a bench above my grave. The manager encouraged me to have a mouse box to mark my spot, but I spent so long trying to get rid of mice from our London flat that this just wouldn't seem right. But I might put a ramp at the end of my bench, from which toy cars can launch into the undergrowth. Gill likes the idea of coming here with the boys, and there are paths leading everywhere. It's not a graveyard in the regular sense because there are no headstones and everything just disappears and becomes part of the wood.

I'm disappearing now, and this above-ground work feels like part of the preparation for the granular changes to come. This *slowing* is probably common to anyone who has the time to really experience dying. It feels like a slight drop in temperature, and in noise too. It's a slowing down, which then gives the appearance that others are moving around much more quickly: Gill, my children, the postman, Frida – my friend's dog. I now have no connection to their speed. It's a gradual introduction to the art of being *still*, not a violent one, as it is for many others. And I think this is something not widely appreciated about my disease: the extent to which it enables a person to gently build up to the moment, as a kind of practice, so that the transition can be made as smooth as possible.

Arrivals

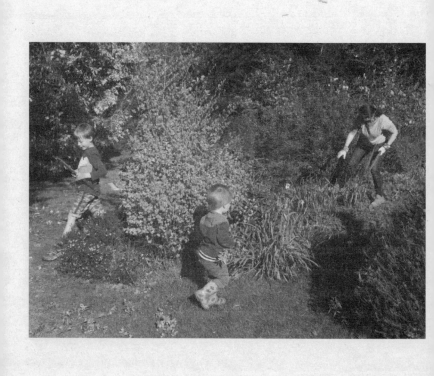

Ten months ago, after first viewing the bungalow, we had crept back on a secret visit to the empty building, skulking around its perimeter, and into a large garden dominated by a vast ash tree. There was another, smaller ash, a little further back, in the wood beyond the garden.

We discovered this woodland, with its deep running brook, accessible from the back of the garden through a broken wooden gate. The trees and water have been described to me, but the land beyond our garden descends to such an extent that, even when we first viewed the bungalow last summer, it was inaccessible with the crutches I was using. On that first occasion, Tom had gone swimming in the brook, as I waited in the grounds of a house we didn't yet own. I remember watching Gill's orange shirt disappearing first, within a green enveloping mass, then Tom, then Jimmy. I watched Tom quietly disappearing into those trees, but he came back as something different, as a child exulted and complete, appearing from behind the green velvet of a conjurer's cloak – mud-splattered from below, dripping from the top, his narrow bare chest pulsing and shivering like a tiny combustion engine, fuelling his motion, rattling his teeth.

For the last five months the bungalow has been a building site, and I've been relying on Tom for progress reports from his Saturday visits with Gill and Jimmy. And with the knowledge of difficulties supposedly common to those who employ builders, it seems remarkable that we have not experienced a single moment of strife and vexation. Instead, our three builders strive away in the background with all the care, attention and devotion of three giant, dusty, leather-handed *mothers*, all working and worrying away – in our absence – on what this building will become. As the months pass, it has become clear that our three giant mothers are not just building an extension for us, but preparing a home; thinking, like any mother would – or three huge, caring, wood-splitting, bricklaying, nail-driving mothers would – of what we will need or want, or what will make us feel just *so*.

It's been my experience that any of us can be a mother when we really need to be, or a father, or whatever we need to be – that being *just* a friend exists at the very beginnings of our imagination. Ten months ago we were collected from Portugal by untold mothers and fathers and, since that time, enough people have held on to us, helping to make sure that we have the home and the support we need. We have been listened to, propped up, encouraged and rescued by virtual strangers and by a few of those we have known almost our entire lives.

For the last five months our home-to-be has been, for me alone, a photographic fiction – comprised of images of Tom and Jimmy eating sandwiches on piles of timber, or wading with wellies through the channels being dug for concrete foundations. The winter leading up to this was the *bungalow season*, marked with a preparatory bungalow weeding and planting party, a bungalow cake, bungalow jokes, bungalow bickering and endless bungalow dreams of different colours and kinds. But now, after sleeping all on top of each other in one stable room, after all this bodily decay, the moment finally arrived when we found ourselves travelling towards the completed building in convoy from the hospice, with Tom and me in the wheelchair taxi, and Gill and Jimmy following behind.

We pulled up and the boys ran straight in, like two ferrets spilled from a hessian sack, but when I reached the big glass doors at the back, and looked out at the giant ash tree at the end of the garden, my body rippled and surged, and some old tide breached upwards and bent me forwards in its flood.

One of the things I've observed is that everyone's face takes on a distinct shape when the tears really come; or at that point of volatile energy just beyond the moment when the tears can no longer be stopped. My own face curls inwards from the sides, and I reach upwards with a paw to a point just above my left eyebrow, as if I'm trying to package up and clear away all the upset before anyone can notice. No matter how far any of us travel in our life, I've formed the theory that our faces in this moment offer the reminder, or the evidence, or the imprint of original feeling. And it makes no difference if these tears come from pain or relief – as these ones did – because our faces have been shaped for these moments back in a distant time in our lives.

Gill had followed me in and her own face cracked open as she bent in around the front of me, across my wheelchair. It's very hard to kiss someone, let alone hug them, when they are reclined in a powered wheelchair. The only way to achieve this is to stretch out like the arterial trunk of a mature tree and to grow around and through the obstacles of a padded armrest or a pro-truding console. Our chests criss-crossed and, within a few moments, my weaker diaphragm had synchronized with Gill's. We carried on like that for what seemed like several minutes.

These were very different emotions to the ones that had surfaced with my friend and beloved uncle, Doctor Tiago, but they seemed to exist at the distinct other end of that time. This bungalow was such a long way from his hydroelectric power plant, but I imagined he might have been there with us in this moment; that he might even have been the one to open the bungalow door to us, with his hand sweeping down under the broad warmth of his smile and extending out to an arm's length as a gesture that we had finally arrived.

And with Gill and I clasped together, like two entwined and wayward branches, he might have moved in behind our broken and bent torsos, nodding as he looked out at the tree, his smile undimmed and undented, holding our bobbing shoulders in his vast avuncular palms; letting all this energy flow with the knowledge and awareness that all great hydroelectric engineers possess.

At this point, and I don't know, but I think Doctor Tiago could have discreetly broken away from us to make a speech to mark this occasion. More than anyone, he would have been able to measure this moment, occasionally glancing outside and gesticulating towards aspects of *nature* when he felt such reference points illuminated the wider thrust of what he needed to say. It wouldn't have been obvious quite who, if anybody, he was making this speech *to*, but with Gill and I crumpled and twisted up in each other, it would have felt right that someone with this authority in our lives would have returned to mark this auspicious change in circumstances by telling our story.

As I knew from the start, he was a man who could have been anything to us – doctor, engineer, uncle. He could have been a person in the desert selling us chilled coconut water, and perhaps that's exactly what he was. There are some people who can be anything. Everyone knows a person like this, detectable from the wide watery lustre of their eyes, and a face acting in complete unison across all its parts, which is something quite rare and unmuddled in a face. It's a moment of good fortune to have such a person in your life at the very time you need them most but, if that's not the case, or if the timing is wrong, it's particularly important to invent them.

And I feel sure, after clearing his throat, that Doctor Tiago would have commenced with his account of meeting this curiously misplaced English couple in his consultation room, and his recollection of our shared experiences with a pin. His tone would have begun lightly, with a cheerful reference to the lopsided nature of my face, and how this had diverted his attention from recognizing the true nature of my condition.

It's likely he would have remarked upon our many subsequent and temporary homes, serving only to highlight the fitting final residence within which we had settled, with its views of the garden and the wood beyond. And finally, deftly combining a measured tone of both sombreness and felicitousness, he would have reminded his absent audience that this new beginning of ours – like so many of life's arrivals – was also an ending; that we had arrived as an embattled family of four but would one day – some years from now – be leaving this place as something smaller, or different, something with all its pieces no longer completely intact.

And after pausing in this moment, drawing back not just his lips but his entire face, to smile with, of course, his customary warmth, I'm in little doubt – knowing Doctor Tiago as I had come to – that the final point he would have wanted to make is that our eventual *incomplete* departure from this place was a fate that, in one form or another, would eventually be shared by himself and everyone then present, and also by everyone who was not.

When my eyes cleared, and after Gill had pulled away, a very different view of the great ash tree became visible. It was mid March, and its stripped, muscular branches dipped and turned in many directions, like the tentacles of a mythical sea beast. I noticed the moss and daffodils encircling its wide base, then glanced upwards to where the thick neck of one main branch formed a crooked joint, and observed, within this knotted mass, the smallest dark pupil of a hole, set in a smooth almond shape of bare wood.

Tom's red T-shirt came into view, and then its colour disappeared behind a large bush. I could see his head moving above the foliage. I looked further beyond, into the leafless wood itself, with the speckled background colour of the sky visible deep within and, now moving across the foreground, Jimmy's blue wellies.

Afterword

14 December 2019

In the beginning I was just a dad who fell over a bit and then couldn't drive the car. Then we had a name for what was happening to me: motor neurone disease. The rest of my physical decline has taken two years and I now write with a camera attached to a computer, which tracks reflections from my pupils. I can use the same device to talk with my synthetic voice. It's obviously slower to use, and has trained me to get to the point, in much the same way that dying has.

In the room next door, as I write, I can hear Jimmy, my two-year-old son, offering to take passengers on a bus ride to various destinations. It's half-term and Tom, my seven-year-old, has wandered out into the garden. He's smiling, looking back at the house, as he points out a squirrel to someone standing inside. There's adult laughter, too. I can hear Gill, my wife, talking with one of my carers.

I'm in an adjacent downstairs bedroom, suspended in a sling that hangs from the ceiling hoist. It's positioned over a bedpan, and my floppy neck is wedged upright between a pillow and a piece of foam. I usually stay here for a while because it also has a view of the garden. It's gusty and leaves are twirling down from an ash tree.

I realise I've been saying goodbye to my family for two years. Always imagining this version of myself, without a voice or moving parts. But now I'm here, I can see that we're all just interested in the same thing: how anxious all these squirrels are as they bury their treasure in the turf. How they keep looking back over their shoulders. And how life just carries on, until it doesn't.

Children walk past spiders' webs all the time and see little things dying. Death is all around them; they know this better than their parents, who have often forgotten. I know I had. But children haven't reached this stage yet. Death and dying can be known. It doesn't stop them laughing at a fart or making an empty crisp packet go pop. There was a moment halfway through my decline when Tom needed to check whether he would die one day. He was wrapped in a blanket on my lap as I confirmed its inevitability. He sobbed and I pulled the sides of the blanket in around him. After a few moments his tears came to an end, and five minutes later he was upside down on the sofa giggling at his toes.

Jimmy was at my bedside a few mornings ago dispensing imaginary ice-cream. I was staring upwards, and I could hear him low down to my right. I opened and closed my mouth to show that I was eating some of the '[va]nilla' on offer but, silent and motionless, I don't know if he noticed, and then I heard him padding away into the next room.

I can't be active in the life of my children. I have to see what the day brings. There was the moment last week when Tom rested his cheek into my upper arm, gently twisted the top of his head upwards against my flesh like a nestling cat, then twirled away. It was a moment that must have lasted five seconds at most but I kept it with me – held on to it – for days, as if I wasn't just making contact, but taking an imprint.

I owe these moments to materials that are both plastic and hollow. To an expanding network of tubing crisscrossing my body: transparent blues and yellows, concertinaed or smooth. The largest gauge of tubing has the central importance of the eastbound M4 heading into London. This is the one swooshing air and oxygen into my lungs, but there are other tiny subcutaneous tubes more like narrow Cornish lanes, trickling a minuscule palliative cocktail just under the skin of my bicep.

The other key thoroughfare is the one delivering sticky beige nutrition through a macaroni-sized tube running directly into my abdomen.

Tubes are now a way of life and, with so many doctors and nurses coming and going, there's plenty of spare tubing lying around. This place is like a fisherman's cottage but with coils of plastic everywhere – in wicker baskets or hanging from hooks. A lot of it ends up in the bath with my two boys. Or it becomes part of Jimmy's marching trumpet band.

When I was diagnosed, my heart broke in different ways, but some of those feelings have softened. It was always the tiny pieces of future that hurt. I'd imagine Gill and Tom and Jimmy unloading shopping, or just being listless together on a Sunday.

But I'm very still with this disease now: I'm an observer, sensing lives happening in other rooms. I hear bottles and cans rattling in plastic bags. I see the rain at three o'clock on a Sunday. All this detail goes by or around me and I see it working. I see three people moving and turning together – and it's no longer breaking my heart. It's just sad and comforting. I didn't expect the end of my life to feel like the future.

I see and hear my family clowning around and I want so much to be in there with them – teaching my children to brush their teeth in the style of a camel. Instead I'm unnaturally still – observing the way their bodies move to express or receive humour. The way a back curves, or a head is thrown back. Watching hands thrust out wide, or even the opposite of such movements. All the infinite expressions. But I'm not clowning around any more; I just see it going on – how ornate it is, how beautiful.

Other losses are simpler and more incremental. Sometimes they are nothing more than adaptation and sometimes, like the loss of my voice, they are devastating. I lost my swallow very quickly. There was a three-week period when Gill made sure I had lots of really nice soups, and that was it. Food was a thing of the past. I've never got over that loss.

I'm fortunate that my ventilator filters out the aroma of most foods, replacing them with a smell like the inside of a plastic bucket. Occasionally smells get through, like roast lamb or the mist that comes from Tom peeling an orange, but mostly I'm assailed by food memories. The most recent is of the yellow Styrofoam containing takeaway from a Lebanese restaurant. Other food memories are more permanent and catastrophic, and these are all the foods I ever made or shared with my young family.

When the boys are in bed, Gill climbs up on to my hospital bed and sometimes falls asleep. It can feel like I've been waiting the whole day for this moment.

Watching Gill asleep always feels like such peace to me, and some of this article would have been written with Gill by my side in that way.

It's really hard to cry when you rely on a mask for air. I use a mask that's attached to my nose, so when I cry my mouth stretches wide open and all the valuable air gusts out, like a badly insulated letter box. And the camera I use to communicate can't track the progress of my pupils, so crying is a form of incapacitation. It's so much easier for Gill, who can stretch out on the bed and sob without any of these secondary difficulties. It's not that we're always crying together. It just happens sometimes. Recently Gill's been reading to me from old travel diaries, written in the days before we had children. Stories of mountains and recklessness on motorbikes, other countries. The past feels so luxurious.

But now it's the present. It's all been leading up to this. Sad but no longer broken. Here with Gill. It's a magical kind of sadness, saying goodbye. A bit like preparing to travel again, but no longer together.

— First published in the *Guardian*.

Acknowledgements

Hundreds contributed to the fundraising that helped return us from the top of a Portuguese mountain, to a settled life back in the UK. I wish I could name everyone.

Those mentioned below have supported family life in unique and imaginative ways. These are all people who noticed us and became the community we needed. They will always be part of our story.

Julia & Ed Banks, Xin & Jessie Zhu, Cinead O'Sullivan, Emma Collins, Paul Edge, Susan Edge, Jason Silk, Leigh Short, Kim Wilson, Sam Goodwin, Kayode Adeniji, Matthew Quint, All staff from ward E6 of Portsmouth's Queen Alexandra Hospital, Roisin O'Sullivan, Mandy & Dennis O'Sullivan, Emma Gilgunn-Jones, Peter Lamb, Simon Lace & family, Lucy Elphinstone, The staff, student & parent community of Francis Holland School (SW1), Natasha Warne, Nicola Morrill & family, Kim

Archer, Ashley Tong, Deborah Gosling, Helen Vickery, Sarah Wolverson, Phil Desmules, Sonja & John Doris, Manjeet & Russ Turner, Kate Fismer, Father Bernhard Schunemann, Mary-Ann Ridgeway, Yasmin Page, The staff & parent community of Inwoods Small School, Sarah Lowson, Mariamah Mount, Emma Ball, Nat Segnit, Louise Morley, Isabel Ferreira, Suzanne Cook, Simon & Victoria Cobden, Brian Sawkins, Heather Woodrow, Ellie Lloyd, Mary Goldberg, Stephanie Tyrer, Stephanie Pattenden, Miranda & Roderick Williams, Joel Cadbury, Orpha Phelan, Phil Williams, Anna Mayer, Tom Macken, Alex & Suz Crichton-Stuart, Elina Borin, Joy Coughlan, Andy Salter, Chris Weitz, Lilita Grinberga, Dan Gent, Guiseppe Rufini, Laura Camfield, Louise Cartledge.